Belinda Grant Viagas, N.D, D.O, Dip. C, trained as a Naturopath, Osteopath and Counsellor and has her own Natural Healthcare practice. She is the author of several bestselling books on natural healthcare, including: *Natural Remedies for Common Complaints*; *Natural Healthcare for Women*; *Detox Diet Book*; and *Stress: Restoring Balance to Our Lives* (The Women's Press, 2001). She works with individuals and groups and travels widely with her programme of lectures and workshops.

Also by Belinda Grant Viagas from The Women's Press:

Stress: Restoring Balance to Our Lives (2001)

SLEEP

A Natural Guide

BELINDA GRANT VIAGAS

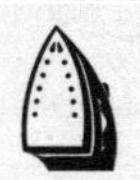

To Nora – with love

This book is not intended as a substitute for professional medical advice. Anyone who has a medical condition, or is concerned about his or her health, is advised to consult with a qualified practitioner.

The authors and publishers cannot be held liable for any errors, omissions, or actions that may be taken as a consequence of consulting this book.

First published by The Women's Press Ltd, 2001
A member of the Namara Group
34 Great Sutton Street, London EC1V OLQ
www.the-womens-press.com

British Library Cataloguing-in-Publication Data
A catalogue record for this book is available from the British Library.

ISBN 0 7043 4632 X

Typeset in 10.5/15 Trump Medieval by FiSH Books Ltd, London
Printed and bound in Great Britain by Cox & Wyman Ltd,
Reading, Berkshire

Acknowledgements

Thanks to Raymond Haris, my favourite ever poet, accountant and gardener – a true Renaissance man! Margot O'Shea blessed me with her networking and tireless organisational skills. Mary Farragher and the team made my days at the office much more agreeable, and I am greatly appreciative of the support and encouragement of the County Library service, especially that of Austin Vaughan and Eleanor O'Toole. Sean and Clodagh McCaughey were there with essential help and support, reason and good dinners. My thanks also to Darragh Hammond of Naturalife, and, for her work editing this book, to Kirsty Dunseath at The Women's Press.

Contents

Introduction

We all sleep, and for some of us it just happens quite naturally at a regular time each evening, or whenever we put our heads down. However most people experience difficulties relating to sleep at some stage in their lives, whether it is an inability to fall asleep at night or to sleep for more than a few hours without waking. Anyone who has ever experienced the sheer despair of tossing and turning all night knows that insomnia is no trivial matter. Some people find it hard to rouse themselves from sleep, and face each morning feeling groggy and sluggish, while others feel tired all the time. Periods of change such as the birth of a baby or the onset of the menopause bring their own challenges.

On average we spend 8 hours in every 24 asleep – a large chunk of time, yet very little is understood about the mysterious processes that go on during this time. Strange things happen while we sleep: we all know of people who go for walks or hold conversations, then waken a few hours later with no memory at all of what they have been doing. During sleep our brainwaves change and our body relaxes. It is also the body's chance to renew itself and repair the effects of the day. The growth hormone responsible for cell regeneration floods the body so that even routine repair work is carried out much faster than when we are involved in other activities. And the mind has a chance to do some housekeeping too, reviewing many of the day's events through dreams, processing new information, and laying down memories.

The events of sleep are fascinating, and can be distinguished into different stages and cycles. At certain points during the night we are prone to disturbance, while at others we are so deep in our slumber that it would be difficult, if not unwise, to stir us. Indeed, in certain societies and cultures it is considered extremely dangerous to wake a Shaman or Wise Woman in case the fabric of their dreams is torn.

An unmet need for sleep can cause tremendous problems. A person who is sleep deprived is more likely to be involved in an accident, be less productive in their work, have poorer social skills and be more prone to negative moods and depression. Lack of sleep will produce some of the same symptoms as long-term exposure to stress, impacting further on our health and our ability to cope with the demands of a busy life. Major industrial catastrophes, such as the Three Mile Island nuclear incident in America, have been attributed to human errors that occurred during the time when the body is generally at its sleepiest.[1] Fatigue is currently blamed for about one-third of all traffic accidents and is more likely to cause road deaths than drink-driving.[2]

Current estimates are that between 25–60 per cent of us are chronically sleep deprived. The National Foundation of Sleep Disorders in the United States found that at least 40 per cent of women and 30 per cent of men have experienced sleep disorders of some kind[3] and a poll by the National Sleep Foundation found that one in two people have suffered from sleeplessness at some point in their lives.[4]

Many of us have been tired for so long that we don't even know it. And yet we continue to raise children, drive cars and get on with our lives. We try to 'catch up' on sleep at the weekends or rely on stimulants such as coffee to get us through the day. But most people are aware of how ineffective short-term remedies can be. What your body really needs is sleep.

In our culture it has become quite a macho thing to say that we don't need much sleep – 'I only need two hours sleep a night and I manage to run a small country on that'. In reality most of us need more sleep than we are getting. Women in particular often have to balance a job and a busy home life, yet a working woman is likely

---

1 Ian Hindmarsh, quoted in *Daily Telegraph*, 28 July 2000
2 *Journal of Occupational and Environmental Medicine*, 19 September 2000
3 http://www.health-alliance.com
4 http://www.sleepfoundation.org

to average around 6¾ hours sleep during the working week, well short of her needs. Simply getting by is not enough when the price we pay is memory loss, lack of physical renewal, low energy levels, general irritability, mood swings and an inability to concentrate.

Much of what we do during the day will influence how well and how much we sleep at night. Being physically weary is a good way to ensure a good night's rest, as is having tied up loose ends, whether they be practical or psychological – one of the worst things we can do is to lie in bed worrying. But a host of other factors also influence our night-times, ranging from the food we eat, and when we eat it, to the layout of our bedrooms and how fulfilled we are in our lives and relationships.

This book is a guide to sleep and the many factors that influence it, some of which may be surprising. It encourages an individual approach, helping us to discover our own sleep needs, and suggests ways of regulating our sleeping habits and patterns, with practical tips on how to improve the quality of our sleep and its quantity. A good night's sleep is a treasure to be valued. It is part of a natural cycle that honours all our needs and enables us to face each day with optimum energy and well-being.

Chapter 1 – The Facts

The patterns of our day follow a clear rhythm and these impact on our sleeping habits. Within every 24 hours, humans, plants, animals and all living things pass through a clear journey of change, during which body temperature will rise and fall, opportunities for sleep will occur, appetite will peak and different organs in the body will become more active. These **circadian rhythms** originate from the time when our activities were governed by the light of the sun and our bodies still respond to them today, even though we rely on other sources of light. For example, we all experience a rise in our body temperature after midday, and it falls to its lowest point between 3 and 5 a.m. We find it easiest to sleep when our body temperature is falling during the late evening, and easiest to wake up in the morning as our temperature rises. Shorter cycles, such as the rhythm of a beating heart or digestion are termed

ultradian rhythms. The patterns that occur within sleep can be defined as ultradian rhythms and tend to have a duration of around 90–100 minutes.

Although sleep is a very basic necessity, we still know relatively little about the mechanics of it, and new discoveries are being made all the time. It was only in 1953, when physiologists Eugene Aserinsky and Nathaniel Kleitman first identified Rapid Eye-Movement (REM), that scientific thinking on sleep really began to flourish. We do know that different parts of our brain are alert at different times during the night, and our understanding of what this means is growing. Studies have also shown that being woken at different stages in the sleep pattern will affect an individual's ability to remember their dreams, and may also be more or less disruptive to the next day's energy levels.

While we are asleep, we have a basic awareness of what is going on around us. This is what enables us to wake in response to a noise, or to someone moving close by. This is also what can keep us awake at night when we have noisy neighbours or when we are sleeping with a new partner.

During sleep our muscles tend to be relaxed, but although the body feels as though it is at rest, there is a significant amount of repair work going on at cellular level. The brain is also involved in various processes as the neurones that transmit messages and account for much of our mental activity are renewed. Recent research, using positron emission topography brain scans, shows that one function of our dreams may be the sorting out and converting of new information into longer-term memory. Scans have shown almost identical readings taken while people were dreaming to those taken the previous day while they were learning a new skill. This suggests very strongly that the brain was running an action replay of the day's events at night.[1] Further research has demonstrated that those learning a new skill will show significantly better results when tested the next day if they have had a night's sleep.[2] This reinforces the theory that sleep not only contributes to the hard wiring of memory, but is also essential to proper, alert functioning during the day.

The Sleep Cycle

Accurate readings of the electrical activity in the brain can be taken by measuring the waves of electrical activity it produces. This is recorded by placing electrodes that are connected to a machine called an Electroencephalogram or EEG onto the head. During periods of extreme excitation, such as an epileptic seizure, the EEG will show very high voltage, synchronous discharges. When we are normally awake and mentally active the machine will record an asynchronous, high frequency, low voltage response – our brain is 'working' relatively quickly. As we begin to relax, the frequency of the electrical waves begins to slow down.

---

1 Neil Stanley, Director, HPRU Sleep Laboratory, Surrey University. Quoted in *Daily Telegraph*, 28 July 2000

2 Rita Carter, 'Ultimate Health Part 3', in *You Magazine*, 18 February 1996

By measuring these waves and observing physical characteristics, scientists have defined two different types of sleep – **NREM** (non rapid eye-movement) and **REM** (rapid eye-movement).

NREM sleep occupies most of the time we spend asleep (about 75–80 per cent), with REM sleep, taking up the remainder. During a normal night, REM sleep follows each of the 4–6 cycles of NREM sleep, with each complete cycle usually lasting between 1½ and 2 hours. Each cycle repeats the same pattern, with sleep gradually becoming deeper then returning to light sleep, possibly followed by a brief episode of wakefulness.

Sleep latency is the period of time it takes us to fall asleep. This can vary considerably. If we are chronically sleep deprived, we are likely to feel as though we fall asleep the minute our head hits the pillow, and our sleep latency could be as little as 3–5 minutes. However the norm is about 20 minutes. During this time we are slowing down, our awareness is shifting, and our body is beginning to relax in preparation for sleep.

Stage 1 of our sleeping pattern is essentially a time of transition. The world seems to be fading into the distance and we are likely to experience changes in the ease with which we recognise sound. This is also when we may experience sudden muscle spasms or the feeling of falling, both of which are symptomatic of the changes in brainwave activity. EEG readings of Stage 1 sleep are characterised by low voltage mixed frequency tracings with a considerable amount of theta waves (4–7 hertz or cycles per second).

Stage 2 sees our brainwaves slowing still further, but with sudden short sequences of waves of 12–14 hertz called 'sleep spindles' and other distinctive waveforms called K complexes. Entering Stage 2 means that our brain has made the commitment to sleep rather than just doze. It may blend into the other sleep stages or last on its own for about 30 minutes but in general it accounts for about 50 per cent of the time we spend asleep. This is the level of awareness that we return to often during the night, and may be when we are 'checking out' the immediate environment for safety as well as doing a fairly thorough inner check to confirm that our body systems are fully functional. If anything important happens we will be able to respond.

Stages 3 and 4 are the deepest levels of sleep, with the brain slowing into delta waves (1–2 hertz). During this time we are very vulnerable to disturbance, but are likely to find it hard to wake up fully if roused. Blood pressure, heart rate, muscle tone and rate of breathing are all reduced. The main difference between Stages 3 and 4 is the amount of delta-wave activity and the continual lengthening and deepening of the brainwaves recorded on the EEG. The figures vary, but together these stages are estimated to make up anywhere between 10 and 25 per cent of overall sleeping time and are often considered to be the most restorative. They are perhaps also when the brain does much of its learning from the events of the day. Certainly children spend a great deal of sleeping time in Stages 3 and 4, assimilating the massive amounts of information they learn each day and facilitating the work of growth hormones. The proportion of time we spend in Stages 3 and 4 reduces significantly as we grow older. It also reduces as the night progresses, with more of our time spent in Stage 2 and REM sleep.

REM sleep occurs near the end of each cycle, and periods of REM tend to increase in length over the course of the night. REM sleep is recorded as low voltage, mixed frequency activity on an EEG. During this time we lose the ability to regulate our body temperature so there is no shivering or sweating, and both our breathing and heartbeat become more erratic. We stop breathing with our ribcage and rely on the diaphragm instead. Another characteristic of this stage is that the body becomes virtually immobile and muscle tone is further reduced, although there may be some twitching of the muscles on the face, fingers and toes. The brain is extremely active, almost like our waking state and brain temperature is increased. Blood flow changes lead to increased vascularity in the sexual organs, which is why we may feel aroused or why men often find they have an erection when they wake. The most obvious physical characteristic is, of course, the rapid eye-movement itself.

Scientists used to think that dreams only occurred during REM sleep but we now know that mental activity continues throughout both types. The experience of dreams, however, seems to be clearer and more profound during periods of REM and if a person is woken during this time they are more likely to remember their dreams. Sleepwalking and night terrors tend to occur during NREM sleep, usually in Stages 3 and 4, and are less likely to be remembered the next day.

While We are Sleeping...

While we are asleep our bodies are involved in the anabolic work of building and repairing, and waking sees us begin a period of catabolic or breaking-down work, ready for elimination and activity. During the day, while we are awake and active, adrenaline circulates through the body. This gives us our capacity to deal with stress or shock by fighting or taking flight – providing us with the speed, strength, and the clarity of mind we need to stay safe. This is also one of the hormones, along with noradrenaline and cortisol, that can cause many stress-related symptoms when we are constantly being over-stimulated by internal or external events. Corticosteroids, which regulate salts, carbohydrates and sexual physiology, work together with adrenaline and interfere with the work of growth hormones. When night-time comes, the levels of these 'activity' hormones drop and growth hormones can direct the body to repair, renew and revitalise itself.

Melatonin is another hormone that is involved in our sleep patterns. It inhibits wakefulness and is released by the pineal gland at night. Levels in the blood reach a peak between 1 a.m. and 5 a.m., making it very difficult to be or to stay awake during this time. It is affected by the amount of sunlight we see and can account for some of the seasonal changes we experience throughout the year. Current research suggests that excess melatonin release contributes to SAD or Seasonal Affective Disorder – the depression that comes on during the winter months, when there is less daylight.

Our fertility hormones affect us too and the influence of the menstrual cycle on sleep patterns is discussed more fully in Chapter 3. In males, testosterone levels reach a peak at around 7 a.m., also influencing wakefulness.

While we sleep neurones and neurotransmitters – the compounds that facilitate message transfer and delivery within the nervous system – are being renewed. The neurotransmitter serotonin is important for initiating sleep, and it is made within the body when there is a sufficient amount of the amino acid tryptophan (see Chapter 6). Our immune system is also refreshed, especially during the deepest stages of sleep. The immune system works best when under the control of the parasympathetic nervous system, which is the part of the nervous system that assumes control when we are asleep and also when we are resting, relaxing or meditating. It is a subdivision of the 'autonomic' nerve system, which we do not consciously control, but which regulates our heartbeat, peristalsis (the way food is moved through the gut), stomach, gland and blood vessel activity.

Growth and Change

During our first few weeks of life, we will spend most of our time asleep, waking every three or four hours for a feed. This type of intermittent sleep pattern is termed **polyphasic sleep**. As we grow up, sleep becomes less frequent until we generally sleep for just one long period at night – **monophasic sleep**.

When we reach our senior years, the pattern of our lives changes considerably, along with the way our body works. With retirement and increased leisure time, the tendency and freedom to nap are significantly increased and the sleep pattern becomes more fragmented, shifting back towards polyphasic sleep with shorter night-time rest. Physical activity tends to decrease and with it the need for restorative sleep. In the current pharmacological culture, the amount of medication we are likely to be taking and our higher susceptibility to degenerative conditions factor heavily.

The composition of our sleep also changes with age. Newborn babies spend as much as 50 per cent of their sleep in periods of REM sleep while adults spend only about 25 per cent, decreasing to less than 20 per cent in the later stages of life. As we age, we tend to sleep more lightly with considerably less time spent in Stage 4 of NREM sleep – this means we are disturbed more easily and may find sleep less restorative. Of course external factors probably play a significant part in these changes too – lack of exercise as well as the lack of a sufficiently stimulating environment and of challenging daytime activity can all influence the quality of our sleep, whatever age we are.

The Effect on our Health

Sleep deprivation impacts upon our health in many ways. Fatigue can impair our normal mental awareness, making us confused or less perceptive and slowing down our reaction times. Some researchers have even made a connection between sleep patterns and diseases of the brain such as Alzheimer's, the degenerative disease also known as senile, or pre-senile dementia. High levels of a protein derived from Interleukin I can be found in the brains of those suffering from Alzheimer's and levels of this protein also increase when we are deprived of sleep, possibly creating a pre-disposition to neurone damage.[3] The complex nature of Alzheimer's is still the subject of much medical research, so we cannot be sure of the extent to which sleep deprivation and such diseases are linked. However Interleukin I levels are also significantly higher after a period of infection, and this may be one of the reasons we feel such a great need for sleep in order to recover from even relatively minor illnesses such as a cold.

Another consequence of sleep deprivation is that we can experience memory lapses. Given the connections made between sleep and the consolidation of memory, it is not unreasonable to assume that insufficient sleep will mean we are less able to build on the events of the day. This has important ramifications for us on all levels, impacting upon the effectiveness of periods of study and our ability to recall information when we need it.

---

3 D Foley, 'Sorting Out Sleep in Patients with Alzheimer's Disease', *The Lancet*, 1999

When our sleep is disrupted or cut short, we lose the restorative benefits that would normally have been gained during this time. Those of us who sleep poorly, or who experience disrupted sleep for long periods, are more likely to have higher blood pressure and higher cholesterol levels.[4] A major cause of sleep disturbance is heavy snoring or sleep apnoea (see p157) and these problems can increase blood pressure and damage the heart because of oxygen debt.

When digestion is upset, because the cycles of the day have become disrupted, we can experience high stomach acid activity at times when no meal has been eaten, and low digestive enzyme activity when there is food in our system. Breathing problems during sleep also disrupt digestion due to the pressure changes they create in the chest, which can suck acid out of the stomach and into the oesophagus or even the lungs. This can result in a painful burning sensation, coughing, and sometimes even permanent damage to the lining of the oesophagus.

One of the worst casualities of poor sleep, and one that is immediately apparent, is our mood. When we are tired, we can feel irritable, unmotivated, emotional, impatient and unable to cope with even small demands. Our mood affects every aspect of our lives, from our personal and professional relationships to our health, so we owe to ourselves to make sure that when it comes to sleep we are getting enough, not just getting by.

---

4 MH Beers and R Berkow, *The Merck Manual of Diagnosis and Therapy*, section 14, chapter 173, 17th edition

Chapter 2 – Getting Enough

The amount of sleep that we need is influenced by a number of factors including our genetic make up, the time of year, climate and where we are in our monthly cycle. During the longer nights of winter our body clock becomes conditioned to enjoying more sleep. This is partly due to the shorter exposure to sunlight, and partly an adaptive response to the cold. When we are exposed to constant low temperatures, our body stores fat more readily, our metabolic rate slows down and our body is slower to heal, so our need for sleep is slightly increased – it is when we come closest to hibernating! Similarly, when we experience a period of much warmer weather than usual, it can be difficult to sleep through the night. We also sleep more when we are ill or fighting infection, because the body has more repair work to do. Getting enough sleep on a regular basis will help increase a person's resistance to infection and enhance their general health.

Before the advent of electricity (which was quite recent in evolutionary terms), we were inclined to get around 10 hours' sleep a night.[1] Today the average length of sleep is between 7 and 8 hours and although some of us will do well on this, many people actually need closer to 9, sometimes even 9½ hours' sleep, to function at their best.[2] Of course, sleep needs vary from one person to another, but most of us simply aren't getting enough. In 1999, a Gallup poll of 1000 people showed that 18 per cent of men had fallen asleep at the wheel, 5 per cent said that sleepiness affected their daily activities and 7 per cent reported that they had visited their doctor with a sleep problem.[3] As mentioned in the Introduction, the United States' National Sleep Foundation has discovered even more worrying statistics – 63 per cent of those polled averaged less than 8 hours of sleep a night, with nearly one-third sleeping for less than 7 hours. The US National Commission on Sleep Disorders estimated that sleep-related accidents cost the American government nearly US$46 billion per year[4] and although figures have not yet been calculated for Britain, the British Sleep Foundation suggests that they could be in the region of £7 billion per year.[5]

---

1 Sally Hargraves, 'Health, Happiness and a Good Night's Sleep', *The Lancet*, 8 January 2000
2 Karine Spiegel, 'The Impact of Sleep Debt on Metabolic and Endocrine Function', *The Lancet*, 23 October 1999
3 http://www.britishsleepfoundation.org.uk/bsf
4 http://www.sleepfoundation.org
5 http://www.britishsleepfoundation.org.uk

Admitting the loss of sleep, or that we need more than we are getting, is a bit of a taboo subject in today's busy world. Many people cite high achievers such as Napoleon, Churchill and Lady Thatcher, who all reputedly thrived on very little sleep, as examples to be followed rather than exceptions to the rule. In the drive to meet all our commitments and achieve everything on our schedule, it is very easy to squeeze the amount of sleep we get. Yet so many minor health concerns and symptoms of mental sluggishness can be greatly improved simply by getting a little extra sleep. It is also important to think about the long-term consequences on our heath – in general, the longer we suffer sleep deprivation, the more extreme our symptoms become.

Many of us like to think that we can catch up on the week's sleep debt by lying in at the weekend, but this is not effective as a long-term strategy. We have only one sleep mechanism, not a different one for the weekends, so it is better to try to maintain a regular pattern. Indeed, when the clocks change in spring and autumn each year we tend to experience drops in productivity and it can take anything up to six weeks to adjust to the new rhythm. Having said that, it is possible to catch up on lost sleep if we have had just a few late nights, and the body will usually respond very quickly. Most of the major cognitive problems associated with sleep debt will recede within about 24 hours of a good night's sleep as long as we are not habitually sleep deprived. If you have had a few late nights, making up approximately one-third of the hours you have lost will be sufficient to put you back on track.

Remember how satisfying it feels to wake up after a good night's sleep? Try getting an extra hour a night – even just for a short time – to see the benefits. Skin quality and appearance show a marked improvement after only a few days. Quick to follow is an increase in mental acuity, visual clarity (yes, you really will be able to see better, look better and concentrate for longer!) and an upsurge in energy levels. For maximum benefit, go to bed one hour earlier than usual, because this is more in tune with your body's natural rhythms. Often when we begin to change our pattern of sleeping we relax and allow our true feelings of tiredness to emerge, so it is possible that you may actually feel sleepier than usual for a while.

Signs of Sleep Debt

If you fall asleep as soon as your head hits the pillow, it is a good indication that you are routinely not getting enough sleep. If you often fall asleep in front of the television in the evening, struggle to get out of bed in the mornings, have trouble concentrating or remembering things, are feeling tired, irritable or stressed out, then you need to get more sleep. You may have other health concerns, such as a deficiency in your diet (see Chapter 6), but improving the quantity and quality of your sleep will impact positively on your whole experience.

Think about the following statements. If any of them are true for you, and especially if you have experienced them often in the last few weeks, then you need to address your sleep habits now:

- I have felt sleepier than I should do
- I have noticed myself taking naps, sometimes unwillingly – just dropping off
- I have slept for more than 9½ hours in a 24-hour period and still not felt refreshed
- I have been unable to keep my attention on something even though it interested me
- I have fallen asleep while watching a programme on television, or at the cinema, or while involved in a conversation
- I have had to work at keeping myself awake – by drinking coffee, opening a window, etc
- I have made errors or mistakes because I felt tired
- I have struggled with fatigue in challenging situations, such as when driving
- I have had to stop doing something I enjoy because of a lack of energy
- I can fall asleep anytime, anywhere.

One of the most obvious and immediate signs of needing to sleep is the yawn. We actually yawn for a variety of reasons – to release static tension in the jaw, to improve diaphragmatic activity and to gain more oxygen. The latter is the most common sleep-related yawn and shows us that the body is in need of more energy. Smokers rob themselves of oxygen and the ability to transport it around their body, so are likely to yawn more than others. You will also probably find yourself yawning in a smoky or dust-filled atmosphere for the same reason.

Frequent yawning may be a sign of imbalance in the body, however, and there are many natural remedies to address this. Coenzyme Q10 can be taken as a supplement to improve the way that oxygen is taken up by the cells, and increasing the iron in your diet will maximise oxygen transport and make up for what women lose each month as a result of our periods. You will find more information on natural sources of iron in Chapter 6.

Owls and Larks

Some of us experience difficulty in falling asleep, while others find it hard to wake up, no matter how early we've gone to bed the night before. These habits can become ingrained, but should respond to change if we are persistent.

A common cause of chronic sleep problems is habitually going to bed later each night. We often do this thinking we will complete just one more task, or do one more job, little realising that the quality of our concentration is waning and that we are setting up long-term problems for ourselves. If this seems familiar to you, and you are tempted to stay up late, focus on the positive benefits that sleep will bring. Prioritising sleep means putting your health needs first.

If you have drifted into late bedtimes over the weekend you will probably find it difficult to shift your time clock back to early nights at the beginning of the week. This is because we normally experience an increase in wakefulness a couple of hours before our usual bedtime, and will therefore find it very difficult to get to sleep at this time.[6] We do not know exactly why this is but it may be a rhythm that evolved when our ancestors needed to be more alert as dusk approached in order to seek out a secure place for the night.[7]

Some of us also appear to have a circadian rhythm that is slightly longer than 24 hours, encouraging us to seek or respond well to an ever-later bedtime. It is worth taking notice of any specific reason why you might be finding it difficult to sleep – are you thinking about tomorrow or your finances? Perhaps you simply feel too energetic to go to bed? Chapter 4 looks at ways of putting the day behind you and winding down to sleep.

Some of us are just night owls and our system will stubbornly refuse any attempt to regulate it. If you have tried to reform your habits and failed (it is always worth trying), just accept defeat gracefully and enjoy the pleasures offered by late nights, such as the amazing panorama of the night sky. Ideally you should look for work that enables you to keep these hours, or seek to balance your day by splitting your sleep time and having a long siesta.

Getting up early can be a real challenge to some, but it also depends on the actual time we choose. The body's organs all go through their own cycles of energy and rest throughout the day and night, and there is a particular slump between the hours of 7 and 9 a.m. If you usually get up at 8 a.m., right in the middle of this

---

6 P Lavie, 'Sleep-Wake as a Biological Rhythm', *Annual Review of Psychology*, 2001

7 Dr Raj Persaud, *Daily Telegraph*, 10 January 2001

period, you will notice a considerable difference if you get up just 30 minutes earlier. Waking before 7 a.m. is likely to be most beneficial, so the more you move out of this time frame the better. At first, you may find that you experience a small decrease in energy around 8–9 a.m., probably closer to 9 a.m., but this can be minimised by avoiding sweet things for breakfast so that you do not further upset your blood sugar levels.

Some people find that they awaken in the very early hours of the morning and are unable to fall asleep again. This can be a sign of anxiety and possibly depression (see p146), or may point to another health concern.

The true larks among us are able to rise early, and express their energy along with the waking of the day. These people seem very much in tune with daylight rhythms, and are usually able to fall asleep naturally at an early hour each evening. Even if this is not your normal or habitual pattern, it is well worth experiencing the early morning because of the quiet expectancy and creativity of this time.

If you share your life and your bed with someone who exhibits the opposite sleep pattern to you, you will have to think carefully about ways to avoid disrupting each other's sleep.

Napping

Naps can be very refreshing and can help us feel more alert. They are best restricted to 20–30 minutes to make sure we do not pass into the deepest stages of sleep from which it is difficult to awake, and which may leave us feeling groggy and dissatisfied, rather than rested. Extended naps lasting for one or two complete sleep cycles, however, can form part of an amended sleep pattern. For example, in the Mediterranean region people tend to sleep for a shorter time at night with a siesta in the afternoon. Mothers often do this too, taking an afternoon nap at the same time as their young children. In cases where there is extreme tiredness – when you are trying to repay a long-standing sleep debt, or when recovering from illness, or while engaged in strong physical exertion – a long afternoon nap can also help you sleep better at night. This seems to work best if you are at the stage where you feel so exhausted that you can hardly make it to bed each night. If this is your experience, napping may be beneficial, but it must not interfere with your night-time sleep and should only be considered as a short-term plan to answer your immediate needs.

'Power napping' is a useful skill to cultivate. It is very different to just nodding off because you are feeling drowsy – it is a short, planned period of sleep that will boost your mental and physical energy levels. It is wise to prepare yourself if you are going to rely on your power nap, because it can take some time to perfect the technique. Pregnancy is an ideal period to start learning this skill as it will help you to prepare for the dramatic changes you are likely to encounter during the first few months of motherhood.

Top Tips for Power Napping

- A power nap is necessarily short. Plan to power nap for 10–25 minutes.
- Choose your location well. Make sure that you will not be disturbed and that the place you have chosen is comfortable. Cover yourself so you will not be cold, and make sure you have something to support your head like a pillow or cushion.
- It may take a while for you to develop the ability to nap, so do not worry if you do not fall asleep – begin by being quiet and relaxed and you will still benefit from the short rest.
- Although the ability to wake up naturally after 20 minutes or so is ideal, it is OK to use an alarm clock and this may be the most effective method while you are still honing your ability to nap.
- Practice makes perfect!
- Plan to give yourself at least five minutes after you wake up in which to reorientate yourself before you get on with your day.
- Don't power nap if it interferes with your main night-time sleep.

Sleeping Well

We need to ensure that we make the time and the space for sleep, and that we prepare for it well. It is very easy to sacrifice sleep in a busy life in which there never seems to be enough hours in the day, but this is just depriving ourselves of something that is essential to our well-being. There are lots of good reasons to want to improve your sleep, from wanting to get rid of minor health concerns, to enjoying the luxury of sleeping right through the night. The sleep we get is affected by the things we have done during the day and will in turn impact upon the things we do the next day. Understanding your sleep patterns and the factors that might be disrupting them is the key to dealing with any problems that you might experience, and will help you find a solution to fit your individual needs.

Chapter 3 – Women and Sleep

Change comes naturally to women. We are closely connected with the natural rhythms of life and experience a phenomenal range of changes each month as we travel through our menstrual cycle. The hormonal variations that occur with menstruation, pregnancy and the menopause impact on everything from our appetite, sexual interest, moods and emotions to our mental clarity, as well as influencing the quality and quantity of our sleep.

We also face many external challenges in today's busy world. Although women's rights have come a long way, we still shoulder an unequal burden in the home, often juggling a full-time job, housework, childcare and the demands of family life. We still have to contend with issues such as unequal pay, the social pressure to look good and varying degrees of discrimination. Mother, lover, wife, homemaker, employer or employee – no wonder many women find themselves unable to sleep at night! The daily pressure to fulfil the roles expected of us and yet maintain a strong sense of who we are and what we want can exert enormous pressure, impacting on our ability to fall asleep at night and to achieve the amount of rest we need.

The Menstrual Cycle

With each monthly cycle we face a potential roller-coaster ride of hormonal activity. Although each cycle can be different, and working out your own individual pattern is the key to understanding your changing energy levels and sleep needs, some hormonal events are predictable.

Pre-ovulation

Our cycle begins with menstruation and many women experience disrupted sleep and increased wakefulness at this time, often linked to other symptoms such as cramps. Levels of the soporific hormone progesterone are lower than at mid-cycle and this may be a contributing factor. We are likely to experience dreams that are more vivid than usual and, however well we sleep, we often awake feeling sluggish and with a heaviness in our limbs. This is probably due less to the fact that our sleep is troubled than to the additional pressure on the spleen. This organ is very important to the smooth functioning of our menstrual cycle as it is involved in the production of new blood cells.

During the pre-ovulation phase oestrogen levels are rising. We tend to ovulate approximately mid-cycle and, if the egg released at this time is fertilised, it will result in pregnancy. If not, the lining of the uterine wall begins to break down and a period follows approximately 14 days later.

Around ovulation energy levels tend to peak and we can find it quite difficult to wind down at night. The body is geared towards conception and what we want most is sex, so that is when this particular remedy will be most useful!

Post-ovulation

As ovulation occurs, progesterone levels begin to increase, reaching their peak on days 18–21 of our cycle, after which they fall. This is a key time to respect the body's reserves of energy and instigate or re-establish a good sleeping pattern, because a few extra hours per night can make a world of difference in the crucial run-up to a period.

It takes a lot of energy to make a period, and getting sufficient sleep at this time enables the body to cope more easily, especially if you tend to experience premenstrual syndrome. The exact causes of PMS are many and varied but falling hormone levels contribute to symptoms such as bloating, moodiness, anxiety, headaches, abdominal cramps and insomnia. If you suffer from PMS try to exercise regularly and avoid caffeine, alcohol and foods high in sugar. Make sure you are eating a balanced diet and in particular that you are getting enough iron and vitamin B_6. Evening primrose oil is a popular remedy to keep energy levels high but there is more of the active compound, GLA (gamma linoleic acid), in borage or starflower oil. Try adding a few fresh borage flowers to a salad or a cool drink. Another wonderful tonic to keep energy levels high and to cope with the mood swings PMS can bring is a cup of home-made fenugreek and molasses tea. Put a tablespoon of fenugreek seeds in 3 cups of water and bring to the boil. Simmer for 3–5 minutes and then strain, discarding the seeds. Sweeten the drink with a teaspoon or so of black strap molasses. You can drink this every other day in the week before your period is due.

Before the advent of electric lighting, women naturally ovulated and bled with the two main phases of the moon. We can still harness this primitive energy today by leaving the curtains open at night and allowing the moon's glow to work on our hormonal balance, but this only works if you don't have street lighting nearby. Traditional wisdom suggests that we will ovulate with the full moon when we are being physically creative, and when we are focusing on inner work, intuition and our spiritual life, we will bleed with the full moon.

Pregnancy

Women are remarkably versatile and resilient. Nature has designed us to birth and nurture our children and so we adapt to the avalanche of changes the birth of a new baby can bring. When you are nursing your baby or caring for a child, you are likely to be woken during the night, perhaps repeatedly. New mothers almost always go through a stage when they feel seriously deprived of sleep, but in time most will establish a different routine to enable everyone to get the amount of sleep they need. Mothers often become accomplished nappers who learn to sleep whenever their baby sleeps. This is not exclusively driven by exhaustion, but is also a sign of our wonderful ability to adapt and the way we bond with our children.

Pregnancy is a time of intense emotional and physical upheaval and it has a huge influence on our sleep patterns, especially during the last few months. In the National Sleep Foundation poll, 78 per cent of women reported more disturbed sleep during pregnancy than at any other time.

First Trimester

In the first few months of pregnancy, women tend to feel more sleepy than usual as our body adapts to all the changes. High levels of progesterone are produced and this increases the drive to sleep. You may feel the need to take more daytime naps than before, especially if your sleep is disturbed at night. As the pregnancy continues, you will probably wake up to urinate more frequently. Some women experience nausea or 'morning sickness' and this can be alleviated by eating something bland like a plain biscuit or cracker.

Second Trimester

This is the honeymoon period! As progesterone increase slows down we are bursting with energy and well-being, and the nausea experienced during the first trimester should disappear. The pressure on the bladder is likely to be less continuous, so you may not wake so frequently during the night.

Third Trimester

The third trimester is when you are most likely to experience disturbed sleep, particularly in the very final stages. The extra weight you are carrying may restrict the movement of your diaphragm and make lying down and changing position uncomfortable. Being full-breasted can be another source of discomfort. Sleeping on an air mattress will reduce the pressure on specific areas by distributing your body weight more evenly and strategic use of pillows can help enormously. Try placing one behind you as you lie on your side to provide support for your back and position another as a soft buffer for your breasts or tummy. A small pillow between your knees will give some relief from tension in the lower back. You can buy pillows specially designed for this that secure around one knee with a Velcro fastening but they can take a little getting used to! If possible, try not to spend too much time lying on your back, as sleeping on your left side allows the best blood flow to the foetus, your uterus and your kidneys. If you experience a lot of back pain, you might consider having a structural check from a chiropractor or osteopath to confirm that your spine is sitting properly.

Waking up during the night because you feel you need to urinate is a very common problem after the second trimester, as pressure is put on the bladder. Not drinking after 7 p.m. will help, but you may find that you need to take an afternoon nap to make up for lost sleep, especially if you are experiencing other symptoms such as heartburn and leg cramps. Make sure you are getting enough exercise during the day and avoid eating fatty or spicy foods.

The good news is that most of these difficulties should disappear when your baby is born. The bad news is that your baby is likely to wake you several times during the night for the first few months, which is why the ability to nap is so important. Where possible, partners or relatives need to devise ways of helping a new mother to get a few extra hours of uninterrupted sleep. Post-natal depression affects 10–20 per cent of women (in fact, several studies estimate that the real figure is much higher), and some researchers believe that a lack of sleep could be a contributing factor. It is a very debilitating condition and can happen at any time in the first year after childbirth, but usually occurs in the first four months. If you think you might be suffering from this, it is important that you tell your healthcare practitioner as soon as possible, because treatment can be effective very quickly.

Babies and Toddlers

Sleep patterns vary widely from one baby to another and it can take up to six months for an infant to learn to sleep through the night. In babies, the ultradian sleep rhythm is half that of adults so their sleep cycles last around 50 minutes. A happy, warm, well-fed and dry baby may sleep through four of these cycles without waking or they may seem to wake, make a few sounds and then fall asleep again.

By about four months old, most babies will sleep for about 14 hours in all, including an average 8-hour stretch. From about six months old, the amount of sleep your baby needs is slowly reduced and many babies will sleep through the night, although they will tend to wake very early in the day – often around 5 a.m.

By the age of one, most toddlers have settled into a sleeping routine that will include one or two naps during the day. By the age of three, most children will only sleep at night but they will need around 12 hours. From the age of six, sleep needs gradually decrease to 10 hours a night and then to the adult average of 8 hours.

There is every reason to keep newborns in bed with you through the night, especially if you are breast-feeding, or a first-time mother, when the anxiety of *not* having your baby close by can keep you awake. There is little evidence to suggest that you will roll over and smother your baby, and much reason to support the deep bonding that occurs if you sleep together and are on hand when your baby needs you. It is also much easier to breastfeed without having to get up. Remember that your baby's temperature will rise from your own body heat, so don't dress them in too many layers, and position your baby on top of your quilt or duvet with their own blankets.

After the first few weeks, you may want to move your baby into a crib in your bedroom or a room nearby. Some cribs have a full drop-down side and are designed to be set up right next to a bed, which may be ideal while you are still breastfeeding.

Your baby's disturbed sleep will wake you – mothers will rise from even the deepest sleep when they hear their baby cry. As well as using a baby monitor, you can now buy devices that register babies' temperatures and the small movements they make during the night. If there is a large change in temperature, or if no movement occurs for a short period of time, an alarm will sound.

When your baby cries, it is worth hovering by for a moment or two as they may fall asleep again in a matter of seconds and picking them up will only waken them fully and disturb their sleep pattern. It is also worth remembering that babies are on a large learning curve and it is our job to educate them well. If we teach them that we always appear the minute they cry, then we are setting up a pattern that could be difficult to break.

Most babies settle quite quickly once their immediate needs have been addressed, but some experience real difficulties. Colic can occur when they are around two weeks old, and this difficult, painful time makes sleeping almost impossible. If you are breastfeeding, your baby may respond well to a reduction in your intake of dairy products, especially cow's milk. Some babies are also less relaxed in the darkness and will benefit from having a dim light left on nearby. But sometimes babies are just grumpy and will not settle. Cranial osteopathy and cranio-sacral therapy (sometimes called paediatric osteopathy) are very gentle practices and are excellent for use on newborns and young children. They can relieve many of the symptoms of distress that children experience because of long or difficult births and are certainly worth considering if your child has had difficulty sleeping from the start. It becomes much harder to resolve sleep problems after the age of two, so it is well worth establishing a good routine as early as possible.

Good Sleep Habits

Children who sleep very little may have inherited or learned this pattern. A lack of physical, mental or emotional stimulation during the day will leave your child with excess energy at night but too much stimulation will also prevent them from settling. Introducing a wind-down routine before bed will help them relax into a good night's sleep, and will instil good habits for later life.

Try to encourage a regular bedtime for yourself as well as your child, and plan a definite time for their afternoon nap. Keep to this routine as much as possible, even if you are away from home. Make sure that the half hour leading up to bedtime is relaxed and calm – this is not the time to let other family members come and play, however exciting that might be. Use quiet music, dim lighting, and your own soothing presence to settle a child and read them a bedtime story or sing a lullaby. Rocking and other repetitive movements are excellent, and some mothers find that playing whale sound or heartbeat recordings also help lull a baby to sleep.

Babies and toddlers who experience sleeping problems can be extremely tiring, and our concern for them, coupled with the shattering effects of our own sleep deprivation, can cause chaos in our lives. Most of us can cope with a few sleepless nights, but an ongoing and relentless period of broken sleep can challenge us beyond measure.

It is worth remembering that children soak up the emotional atmosphere very easily, and can manifest their anxieties through wetting the bed, waking up in the night and other sleep disturbances. Do check that they are feeling safe and secure and try to talk about any issues that may be going on within the family, even if your child is very young. Just use language that they can understand.

Truly hyperactive children are rare but, once diagnosed, they do need to be treated in a special way. You may have a very intelligent child who needs to be stimulated, and all children respond well to dietary change – removing food colourings and other artificial and chemical additives, as well as reducing the amount of sugar they eat will all have a positive effect. If you suspect your child would benefit from special attention consult a natural healthcare practitioner for more advice.

Menopause

Hormonal changes during the menopause are a common cause of sleep problems, and few of us will get through this time without some night-time disturbance. These can be minor and quite comforting – sensations of radiating warmth – or more extreme and unsettling. Hot flushes are caused by decreasing levels of oestrogen and can make you feel like you are on fire. They are usually accompanied by sweating and are a clear signal of the imbalance that occurs as our body changes.

Make sure your bedroom is cool, but not too cold or your body will be trying harder to keep itself warm, and try to use only cotton nightwear and sheets. Minimise any alcohol and don't eat hot, spicy foods such as mustard or chilli during the evening. Keep a saucer or small dish by your bed containing an aromatherapy mix of 2 drops each of peppermint and geranium essential oils, in at least 5 tablespoons of almond, apricot kernel or olive oil. Dab this onto your pulse points before you go to sleep, and rub some gently into your temples. Also keep a glass or jug of water by your bed to sip if you wake with a sweat and a piece of cotton fabric to use as a compress. Placing it over your forehead or on the back of your neck should give you instant relief and will help you to settle again. Make sure you keep the two containers far apart – you do not want to end up drinking your essential oil! Schedule naps or a siesta into your day if you find you aren't getting enough sleep at night.

Herbs are a wonderfully effective treatment during the menopause, but it is always best to get a personal prescription. There is much to suggest that the symptoms we experience are due more to a tired and often nutritionally deficient body than to particular hormonal changes, so it is important to get your health history checked out in order to find the right remedy for you. In general terms there is a lot you can do to relieve the symptoms – choosing soya and other foods that are rich in phyto-oestrogens will help, and eating four brazil nuts a day will provide enough of the mineral selenium to help relieve some of the discomfort of hot flushes. A daily cup of mild sage tea is also effective, as is prioritising quality nutrition.

Emotional Health

As adult women we have the capacity to play, to express ourselves, be creative, communicate, display our courage, feel emotions, accept and act upon our own intuition. We are sexual, sensual beings with the ability to birth and nurture, with imagination and intelligence, and with a strong affinity to nature's own cycles and rhythms.

In our busy lives we often focus on specific aspects and the 'rest' of us gets squeezed in here and there. Sleep is one thing that often comes low on our list of priorities. But it is also important that we attend to our mental and emotional health as well as that of our physical body. Faced with the expectations and stereotypes around femininity, it can be hard for us to articulate our own experience and show our true feelings. Expressing our whole selves, our vulnerability and our strengths, our fears and our pleasure, is vital to our well-being. Repressed emotions can surface at night while we try to fall asleep and are unlikely to help us achieve the rest we need. When we take responsibility for the nurturing and care of others, we must also be sure to look after ourselves.

To feel fulfilled you need to challenge yourself and be open to the possibilities the future might hold. When you discover your own needs you can flex all the muscles of your being. Sleep will come more easily and it is the perfect way to balance and integrate your life.

Chapter 4 – Winding Down to Sleep

There is a lot we can do to enable us to sleep well at night. The patterns of our day influence both how tired we feel and the amount of sleep we need. Making sure that we get good exposure to sunlight at the beginning of the day will help us to establish a good sleeping/waking rhythm, and exercise will tire out us physically, while a stimulating day will ensure that we have exercised our mental faculties.

Beyond balancing our waking life, a wind-down routine that is clearly defined and practised regularly is one of the best possible approaches to a good night's sleep. It is also an excellent way of marking the transition from one phase of our day to another. This means setting a time for going to bed and one for getting up, and sticking to them.

Ayurveda, the natural healthcare practised in India and much of Asia, translates loosely as 'the science of life'. It focuses specifically on the cycles and patterns of energy a body goes through each day (the circadian rhythms) and identifies the times when we can maximise the benefits of activity and rest. According to this system, the best quality sleep comes before midnight and 10.30 p.m. is the optimum time to go to bed. Once you miss this window, you may not catch another wave of sleep until around 1.30 a.m. Try going to bed at one of these time slots (preferably the earlier one) to see if sleep comes more easily to you.

Taking a short walk as night falls is a wonderful way to start the body's gradual relaxation. It is important to change gear as you prepare for sleep, so make the hour before bed a quiet and gentle time when you don't do anything too stimulating or invigorating. Many people enjoy reading but it is important not to choose anything too dense or work related – pouring over the accounts is no way to relax! Don't watch exciting television, go for a run or eat a large meal late at night because all of these activities require time to wind down from afterward. Exercise increases body temperature and heart rate, both of which will affect your ability to fall asleep, so it is best if you plan to exercise early in the day, or at least 4 hours before you sleep. The only exception to this rule is sex. Satisfactory sex, whether exciting or comfortable, is one of the best ways to prepare for sleep.

Make sure to avoid substances that will interfere with your sleep, such as caffeine, nicotine and alcohol. Ideally you should not drink coffee or any caffeine-rich drinks after 2 p.m. and nicotine will also take a few hours to leave your system. A small amount of alcohol such as a modest nightcap or a glass of wine with your evening meal may help relax you, but more than that will rob you of the quality sleep you need in order to recover from its effect on your system.

Begin to focus your energy inward as you prepare for bed. This is the ideal time to write in a journal, indulge in treats such as an aromatherapy bath, share a massage with your partner, or practise your favourite relaxation technique. The best wind-down routines are extremely simple, but regular – the key is in the routine. As you repeat what you do each night, be it meditation or simply a few gentle stretches before bed, your body will begin to associate the pattern with sleep and respond to the cues.

Keeping a Journal

Sometimes our brains just don't seem to slow down at night. We lie in bed fretting over the problems of the day, worrying about the future or concerned about those close to us. One good way of setting issues aside is to make a list of the things you have to do the next day so that you can be sure you won't forget anything. Another is to write down your problems along with possible solutions. It doesn't matter if none of these solutions seem quite right at the time – simply recording them will help you to feel that you are responding actively to difficulties rather than letting them overwhelm you.

It is important to tie up the loose ends from the day's events as much as possible so that you are not carrying any feelings of distress with you into your night's dreaming. Keep a journal by your bed so that you can review your day on an emotional level, recording your inner thoughts and feelings. It is also good to think up some rewards for yourself at this time, focusing on the things you most enjoy, and noting down goals you would like to achieve. Your journal is a great place to pat yourself on the back and acknowledge your accomplishments through the day, whether they are large or small.

In a busy life, it is all too easy to feel burdened by the things we need to change or the responsibilities we bear. Focusing on the positive aspects of our experience – the things we can feel grateful for and what we have already achieved – is a very constructive step and can enhance our emotional health and feelings of well-being. It may be that you have to think for a while before you can uncover anything in your day that you feel thankful for, but it can be a rewarding process, helping us to explore the connections between our inner life and the people and places that surround us.

Treating the Senses

Listening to restful music is a wonderful way to wind down from the day. Some people use motivational tapes to improve the quality of their sleep or to work on another aspect of their life. These tapes usually consist of a number of spoken statements or affirmations that are repeated and are often accompanied by relaxing music. The point is not to listen too hard, but to relax, let your subconscious do the work, and to enjoy the soothing sounds.

We can treat the whole body through our sense of smell too. There are specific aromatherapy oils that can be used if you are experiencing sleeping difficulties (see below), otherwise just choose the scents you enjoy. Do not be surprised if you find yourself picking something cooling, such as peppermint or fennel. Sometimes we need to be warmed and soothed in order to sleep well; at other times we need to feel refreshed. Let your body be your guide.

Essential Oils

- **Lemon grass** is good at settling the body and also the mind. It is a good choice if you feel slightly 'spaced out' or if your thoughts seem to be running too fast.
- **Clary sage**'s distinctive perfume will influence your dreams as well as relaxing your muscles. It is also effective in encouraging the flow and regularity of the menstrual cycle. Do not use this oil earlier in the day, before driving or operating machinery, or if you have taken alcohol.
- **Sandalwood** is a warm and woody scent that is calming and will help allay fear or anxiety. It is especially good for mature skins and will help strengthen and support the kidneys.
- **Ylang Ylang** is a wonderfully heady scent that is also a strong aphrodisiac.
- **Frankincense** or olibanum (oil of Lebanon) is a

superbly rich and comforting oil that will make you feel rejuvenated as well as relaxed.

- **Rose** is a powerful uterine tonic that can soothe and calm and is especially good for settling your emotions.
- **Jasmine** is a marvellous antidepressant with a strongly sensual perfume.
- **Geranium** is naturally uplifting. It will help regulate hormone levels as well as calming your mood and balancing your body.
- **Lavender** is very popular with some people as an aid to sleep, but try using a small amount of it during the day first because it can be quite stimulating.
- **Neroli** and **orange blossom** are often recommended but some find them challenging, especially those of us who are sensitive or experience allergies.

Responses to essential oils may vary throughout our cycle, and with the changing seasons. During the winter, warmer, smokier oils are often favoured, while during hot weather we tend to seek something lighter and cooler.

Do not use any essential oils if you are pregnant without consulting your practitioner first, as some oils are contraindicated during pregnancy. These include basil, cinnamon, clary sage, clove, cypress, fennel, hyssop, juniper, marjoram, myrrh, oregano, rose maroc (bulgar) and thyme.

If you do not have a special burner, try sprinkling 2 drops of your chosen oil on to a handkerchief or your pillow slip (the oils may stain so it is best to use something old), or add them to a warm bath half an hour before you go to bed. Drizzle a few drops of orange blossom over a damp flannel and hang it over the radiator in your bedroom to fill the air with its soothing scent. You could also try wiping your light bulbs (when switched off) with a cloth that has been soaked in a dilution of clove bud oil or rose and enjoy the fragrance as the bulb heats up and disperses it into the room.

Herbs and flowers retain their essential oils when dried and it takes only a gentle warmth to release their aroma. Many commercial herb pillows are based on hops and some people, particularly those with a yeast intolerance, find these irritating. You can make your own sachet from a strip of fabric and a selection of dried flowers or herbs. Consider lavender, rose petals, cloves, lemon balm, verbena, thyme and rosemary. Camomile flowers are especially relaxing, and woodruff is a great aid to sleep.

Place your herbal sachet beneath your pillow and the warmth from your body will be enough to release its scent throughout the night. You can reinforce and unify the effects of your chosen blend by placing further sachets in your wardrobe or drawers, or by using the mixture as pot-pourri in your bedroom.

Relaxation

Being relaxed means that you are better equipped to respond to the events of your life and feel in control. Relaxation is something that we can all learn and it has a cumulative effect, so the more you practise it, the better you get.

The 'relaxation response' is a specific set of circumstances that you can create within your body and it is the direct opposite to the stress response with which we are all too familiar. As the body relaxes:

- The heart rate is reduced
- The heart beats more effectively
- Blood pressure is reduced
- Blood is shunted towards the internal organs, especially those involved with digestion, and digestive enzyme secretions are increased
- The breathing rate slows as oxygen demands are reduced
- Sweat production decreases
- Blood sugar levels are normalised.

Relaxation skills are important not only because they help us sleep, but also because they make us less prone to stress and anxiety-related disorders. Learning to relax can help us cope better with physical discomfort and emotional upheaval, and when we are fully relaxed we experience many of the benefits and sensations of sleep itself. Indeed, deep relaxation may take the place of sleep when there is no alternative, such as when we are travelling or when we have a new baby. It is only a short-term measure, however, as both the mind and body need the restorative processes that only sleep can bring.

If you know that you find it hard to relax physically, the first thing to do is to make sure that you have taken enough exercise or been sufficiently active during the day. Then concentrate your efforts on learning some good relaxation techniques and incorporate them into your wind-down routine at the end of the day. These might include some form of gentle stretching such as yoga or the soothing rhythmic exercises of tai chi. Sitting on the floor for a few minutes and practising deep breathing will be enough to ground some people after a hectic day. A few simple techniques – progressive relaxation, relaxed breathing, 'switching off the lights' and 'stretching out' – are suggested below.

The neck is a prime spot for holding tension, so relaxing this area before you get into bed can be very beneficial. A neck stretcher is a wooden or metal structure, shaped into a gentle curve that you lie on to ease out tension in the neck muscles. As usual, try before you buy because some neck stretchers can feel hard and uncomfortable, and many are designed for men which means they are bigger and have a longer curve that will not fit women's smaller cervical (neck) bones.

Individuals vary and some people find that if they experience a deep sense of relaxation too close to their bedtime, it actually delays them falling asleep. You will need to find out your own level of tolerance and may also discover that you have to develop different techniques for winding down to those you use during the day, as your body might associate the latter with staying awake.

Progressive Relaxation

This is one of the most popular techniques for producing the relaxation response. It works very simply by contrasting tension with relaxation, and involves working through the whole of the body in succession, first tensing it and holding that tightness for a moment or two, then relaxing it and enjoying the sensations of warmth and heaviness. Progressive relaxation can be done at any time and is an excellent introduction to relaxation skills. You can do this sitting up in a comfortable chair or in bed as preparation for sleep.

Begin by contracting the muscles of the face and neck. Hold this for a few seconds and then relax. Take a deep breath before moving on to the next body area, and exhale. Now tighten the muscles of the upper arms and chest, hold for a few seconds, and then relax. Take another deep breath, enjoying the sensation of calm and move on. Work through the lower arms and hands, the abdomen, bottom, thighs, calves and feet. If you are doing this in bed, you might like to single out smaller body areas or muscle groups and really take your time working through the whole body. If you are still feeling tense when you reach your toes, return to your head and start the whole process again.

Relaxed Breathing

We all breathe all of the time, so quite naturally we assume that we are doing it just fine. Our breathing is often tense and shallow, however, and is not as effective or as relaxing as it could be. Ideally, each breath should be able to gently mobilise the shoulder area and relax the neck muscles as well as giving us an internal 'mini-massage' as the diaphragm moves up and down within the body.

Place one hand on your upper chest, just below your neck and position the other on your belly underneath your navel. Relax and breathe normally. If your breathing is shallow, you will find that the hand on your upper chest is moving up and down, while the lower hand will move if you are breathing in a deep and relaxed way. Use these two hands as markers to help you redirect your breath and relax your body. Once you get used to the feeling you will be able to do this without using your hands.

A variation of relaxed breathing is to imagine each breath leaving your body through the soles of your feet, feeling it travel down through your body, carrying away any tension or anxiety as it leaves.

'Switching Off the Lights'

This is a lovely technique that is especially good for helping you get off to sleep. Take some easy, relaxed breaths, and then start working your way through your body from the top of your head down to your toes. At each place you visit, use your imagination to do something symbolising going to sleep, such as turning off the light there. Take your time with each location, allowing yourself at least two or three deep, full and relaxed breaths per image. People often don't get to their feet before nodding off while doing this exercise, and that is fine, or you may like to start at your feet some nights in the interest of balance.

'Stretching Out'

The following routine can be performed extremely slowly to stretch out the muscles and relieve any postural tensions that have accumulated during the day. Remember this is a gentle routine, not exercise, as too much energetic movement is likely to make you feel more awake.

- Begin by standing on the floor with your feet shoulder-width apart. Take a deep breath, and as you breathe out, reach up over your head with your left hand as far as you can. You should feel a gentle stretch all the way down the left side of your body. Now breathe in and lower your left arm. As you breathe out reach up with your right hand, feeling the stretch down your right side. Continue this pattern of relaxing each arm while you breathe in, and then stretching gently when you exhale. Keep all your movements soft and gentle and very slow.
- Clasp your arms together in the air above your head and breathe in. As you breathe out turn your palms upwards and stretch gently towards the ceiling. Make sure to keep your head facing forward, or look down slightly and don't arch your back. If you have any lower back problems, the best way to do this stretch is to gently bend your knees and

stabilise your pelvis by tensing your lower abdominal muscles.

- Now take another deep breath in and as you breathe out let your clasped hands travel a few inches over your head to the right, so that you feel a gentle stretch down the left-hand side of your body. Take another breath in, and this time as you breathe out let your hands move back over to the left and enjoy the gentle stretch down the right-hand side.
- Let your arms fall softly to your side. Now rotate your shoulders backwards three times in a large circular motion, first one, then the other, then both together, breathing normally the whole time.
- Next take a gentle hold on opposite wrists, and hold your hands about 6 inches in front of you, in the middle of your chest. Take a deep breath in, and as you breathe out move your arms around to your left, turning your upper body and head ever so slightly so that you are still looking at your hands. Breathe in and return to the centre. Then breathe out and take your arms round to the right. Repeat this exercise a few times to each side. Be careful to keep your hands at the same distance from your body and do not travel too far – the aim here is *not* to work your muscles hard but to gently stretch out the middle of your body, so you should never feel any burn or discomfort.
- Now rest your hands down by your sides. Take a breath in and as you breathe out, drop your chin

down onto your chest and roll down your whole spine, keeping your legs straight but letting your upper body and arms drop gently towards the ground. Do not pull or stretch, just relax. Linger there for one full breath. Take another breath in, and as you breathe out, slowly and gently roll back up through your spine until you are standing up straight again, lifting your chin off your chest last.

- Now reach down and take hold of your left ankle with your left hand as you breathe in and with your out breath draw your foot up behind you till it is touching your bottom. You should feel a gentle stretch in the front of your thigh. If you feel unsteady, hold on to a door handle or a piece of furniture with your other hand. Hold this gentle stretch for a full breath, then slowly release your foot and let it return to the floor. Repeat with your other foot.
- Take another deep breath in and as you breathe out stand up onto your toes. Repeat this slowly two or three times, feeling the stretch in your feet and through your legs. Next lift up your toes so that you are balancing on your heels. You will not be able to lift very far, but should feel a nice stretch down the back of each calf muscle. Repeat this once or twice, then relax and take a few easy breaths.
- Do a body scan to see if there are any areas that still feel tense – if there are, try gently stretching them again. If you feel fine, stand with your feet slightly apart and bend your knees slightly so that they are not holding any tension. Let your arms hang very

loosely by your side and start a very slow, gentle, twisting movement, swinging your arms loosely from side to side and shifting your weight from one foot to another as you move. Keep this easy and flowing. Breathe well and stay relaxed.

Once you have found a relaxation technique that suits you, try to perform it as regularly as possible until your wind down to sleep becomes second nature.

Meditation

Meditation is a state somewhere between relaxation and sleep and is a wonderful gift to the self. It is an opportunity to experience the seamlessness of one's life and can bring myriad benefits in terms of our physical, mental and emotional health.

During meditation our body is still and relaxed, and our brainwaves move in a pattern similar to the slow waves exhibited during sleep. We do not dream while we meditate but neither is our mind alert to, or responding to, the stimuli that surround us. Meditation is a state that can influence sleep in that it comes very close to mimicking some of its effects. When we meditate regularly the quality of our sleep changes. We are less likely to feel drowsy during the day and will usually fall asleep more easily at night. It can also change the amount of sleep we need – people who meditate regularly often need less. If you are not able to sleep for any reason, then a period of meditation can be almost as refreshing.

There is a natural elegance to the experience of

meditation that makes all the words we might use to describe it seem clumsy. It is a state of being that is so close to our essential nature that words and ideas seem inappropriate. It is a way of being still at the very centre of the fast-spinning wheel of life, and yet not divorced from reality, but more fully involved in it. In the East meditation is considered to be a fundamental aspect of spiritual training and there have been many illuminating texts written about it. One of these, a great source of inspiration to me, is reprinted here. Suspend your critical faculties while you read this, and just reach for the essence of the message:

> Wanting nothing,
> with all your heart,
> stop the stream.
>
> When the world dissolves,
> everything becomes clear.
>
> Go beyond
> this Way or that Way,
> to the farther shore
> where the world dissolves
> and everything becomes clear.
>
> Beyond this shore,
> beyond the farther shore,
> beyond the beyond,
> where there is no beginning,
> no end.
>
> Without fear, go.

Meditate.
Live purely,
be quiet.
Do your work with mastery.

By day the sun shines,
and the warrior in his armour shines.
By night the moon shines,
and the master shines in meditation.

But day and night
the man who is awake
shines in the radiance of the spirit.

Gautama the Buddha, 2500 B.C.

Meditation can have a profound influence on sleep, so start by meditating only in the mornings rather than last thing at night and aim to give yourself between 20 to 45 minutes. More experienced meditators often like to meditate twice each day, once when they awake and then again in the evening. This can give a sense of completeness, rounding out the cycle of the day.

There are said to be 5 basic requirements for successful meditation (these are also the results of regular practice):

- the body needs to be comfortable and still
- the internal energies need to be in balance
- the mind needs to remain focused and not be seduced by thoughts or allowed to wander
- the heart needs to be at peace
- you need to wait patiently, and without expectation.

The most important thing is that you come to meditation with an open mind, and are prepared to connect with your inner being.

You will find meditation easiest if you keep your eyes closed and your body upright but relaxed. Eastern adepts choose either a kneeling position, sitting back on their heels, or the classic yoga position of crossed legs with the feet resting on the upper thighs. If you feel comfortable just sitting in a chair, that is fine too. You could also try kneeling on the floor with a cushion between your bottom and your calves. Check that the very base of your spine is tucked underneath you, your waist is held back, your ribcage is lifted, and your sternum or breastbone is raised, with no tension in your neck or shoulders. This will keep your spine straight. The easiest way to release tension in the neck muscles is to draw your chin back a little.

Rest your hands in your lap or on your thighs and open out your hands so that they are facing palm up.

As you enter meditation, there are many techniques you can choose from in order to steady your mind. People who respond well to a visual stimulus often look at an obvious shape or a brightly coloured symbol for a long time so that it will remain in their mind once they have closed their eyes. Others focus on a chant or sound. Alternatively you can just sit still and attend to your breathing. You might like to begin your meditation by registering those things you are aware of around you – the temperature of the room, the sounds and smells. Thoughts will come to you, images appear, feelings and sensations arise from your body, but the aim is to remain in that part of you that can witness these comings and goings and not travel with them. It is a time when you can see emotions and feelings clearly but not be swept up by them; a period of intense physical awareness, when you *know* that you are much more than your physical body.

You may have to set an alarm to tell you when your meditation time is over or you may just reach a point when you are ready to stop. When this time comes, don't rush – give yourself time to make the transition from your inner world to the practical, everyday outer world. Take a few more relaxed breaths, and focus once more on your senses – the sounds in the room and the feelings in your body. Open your eyes slowly and wait a few moments before moving or getting up. Try not to touch your face or your head for a few minutes.

Regular meditation can bring moments of peace and calm that help us to discover our true needs. When our centre is in harmony, everything that flows from it is too.

Massage

Massage is a gloriously peaceful way to ease away the cares of the day. It is especially stimulating to the body's eliminative channels and a useful way to detox during the spring and autumn, which are traditionally the best times. If you have a partner you might take turns at giving each other a massage on alternate nights as this is a lovely way to increase intimacy. Although the aim is relaxation, you may find that it stimulates you towards love-making and this is fine too. If you are not in a relationship, self-massage will not only soothe your tired muscles but will also answer your skin's real need for touch.

If you are going to use oil, find a way to warm it first so that it will spread easily and won't be a shock to the skin. You can pour some into a bowl and stand it on the radiator for a while, or place it on top of a hot-water bottle that you have covered with a small towel. You never need very much oil, so pour out only a small amount.

Take a little oil and spread it all over your hands, as though you are washing them with soap. Then rub in a little extra and begin to smooth it over the body part you are going to work on. When massaging another person, make sure that your touch is light and sensitive. There are many points on the body where too deep a pressure will be unpleasant or may even cause injury, including the breasts, neck and throat, and the back of the knees.

All parts of the body benefit from being massaged gently, but it does take time to cover the whole body so you might decide to focus on just one area. A back massage gives you a wonderfully broad canvas on which to work and includes that key stress point, the shoulders. Other good suggestions include: a very light massage of the abdomen, especially during and after pregnancy and before your period is due; the feet, which can be every bit as good as a full body massage; or the hands and head.

The real secret to good massage is to let your hands lead you and to relax. Explore all the bumps and hollows, smoothness and textures that you find. Let your hands fall into the soft padding of big muscles and gently trace the outline of bony areas with your finger tips. You can use long, sweeping strokes on wide expanses of flesh and small circular touches around joints. Use gentle pressure if you feel that there is some tension that will give way to you, or just concentrate on pleasuring the skin.

When massaging another person remember to:

- make sure that they are warm enough. If they feel cold they won't be able to relax. Cover body areas that you are not working on, even if the room is warm. Remember that you will feel warm because you are moving and working;
- check that they are comfortable – staying in one position for any length of time can cause muscle tension. If they are lying on their tummy, make sure that you remind them to turn their head from time to time in order to relax the neck muscles. (Full-breasted women may also benefit from a cushion placed under the upper chest.) If they are lying on their back, relieve any postural tension in the lower spine by placing a cushion or pillow underneath their knees;
- be sensitive to any areas where your touch may be unfamiliar or unwelcome;
- never pour oil or squirt cream directly onto

someone's body during a relaxation massage. If it is too warm or too cold, or runs everywhere, you will destroy the sense of calm and the body's trust;

- if you are using essential oils, make sure they are fully diluted (3 drops of essential oil is plenty for a full body massage), and avoid sensitive areas such as nipples, genitals, eyes, and any areas of broken skin that could be burnt or made painful by contact with the oil;
- consider using talcum powder rather than oil or cream if the body or body part is particularly hairy;
- stay relaxed. You convey so much through your hands and the quality of your touch, and it is likely that the recipient of your massage will be especially sensitive to this type of communication. Ensure that the silent messages you give them are not associated with stress or tension.

Massage can be a truly loving and generous experience whether you are communicating your good feelings to yourself or to a partner. It is the perfect antidote to a stressful day and will leave you feeling relaxed and at peace.

Further Needs

There is a lot we can do to ensure a good night's rest in addition to a good wind-down routine. The food we eat and the environment we sleep in all impact on our ability to sleep well and these will be discussed in Chapters 6 and 7. Sometimes, however, we need a little extra help. There are many types of sleeping pill available but these tend to have a negative effect on our health and can be quite addictive (see pp132–35), so it is worth considering the range of natural alternatives that can help us through difficult times.

Chapter 5 – Natural Remedies

Sometimes, no matter what we do, we can't seem to get off to sleep. Perhaps we are going through a very stressful time, such as upheavals in our home or work environment. Worries about children, relationship difficulties, financial problems or health matters can unsettle us and even if we have honed our wind-down technique to perfection, we may feel in need of a little extra help.

If you have already looked at all the other areas of your life that might be affecting your sleep, you might want to consider one of the natural remedies listed below. Bear in mind that most of these remedies are for times when you are experiencing particular difficulties and are not an alternative to establishing a good long-term sleep pattern.

Herbal Remedies

We have already looked at some of the wonderful ways that herbs can enhance and encourage sleep when you add their essential oils to your bath, or warm them to release their medicinal values and fragrance into your home. The most common way of taking a herbal remedy to insomnia is as a tincture, a tablet or in a syrup. You can buy these remedies from your healthcare practitioner – in this way you can be sure they will be of good quality, fresh and effective – or from a health food shop. If you are buying a remedy, Potters is an excellent brand and many shops now have trained staff who will be able to advise you.

The beauty of taking a herb, or a herbal remedy, is that you know you are taking a natural substance that is in balance with the environment and will encourage the most simple and effective form of healing. Although many pharmaceutical drugs are based on herbs and other plants, chemists have isolated what they consider to be the most active part and have synthesised it before mixing it with whatever chemicals they need to stabilise the drug in its final form. When you take the herb or plant itself you get all of the benefits along with nature's built-in safeguards in amounts that are effective and also gentler on your system.

Be sure that you always read the instructions carefully or that you get advice from your practitioner on the dosage you need. Herbal medicine is a powerful and effective tool and it is important that you observe the guidelines and use it wisely.

Here are just a few remedies you might try:

- Passiflora tincture – take these drops regularly about 30 minutes before bedtime and their cumulative effect should be felt after only a few days.

- Hops tea – make this remedy by steeping 3 hops heads in a mug of boiling water for 3–5 minutes, then sip the tea slowly. Some people are allergic to hops, so try this remedy during the day first and take only a small amount. You will know if they trouble you because symptoms will appear as soon as you come into contact with them, such as sneezing when you first open the packet or irritation when you touch them.
- Stand 1/2 oz of valerian in a glass of cold water for 24 hours, and take 1 tablespoon of the liquid on the hour for 3 hours before bedtime.
- Add 1 tablespoon of each of these dried herbs, or a small handful of fresh ones, to 1 pint of cold water: red clover heads, shredded lettuce, and hops or valerian or camomile flowers. Heat this mixture and bring it to the boil, then boil rapidly for 2 minutes. Turn down the heat and simmer for another 2 minutes, then remove from the heat, cover, and leave to cool. After 3 hours, strain the liquid and bottle it. Keep it in the fridge, or in a cool, dark place for up to 4 days and take a small glassful at night. Sweeten to taste with honey if you like, but do not reheat.

You can of course use herbs as aromatherapy (see pp47–8). Here are some particularly useful remedies:

- Tie some juniper berries, a bunch of fresh rosemary and a sprig of lavender or some orange peel or linden flowers in a cotton handkerchief and add to a warm footbath. Soak your feet in the infusion until the water cools.

- Add a camomile teabag or 2 teaspoons of dried camomile to 1 of meadowsweet and 1 of lime flowers, and mix in one teaspoon of grated valerian root. Wrap these herbs in a handkerchief and attach it to the tap of your bath. Let the water run through the herbal blend and then leave the bundle in the bath while you soak. If you cannot get meadowsweet or lime flowers use oats instead.
- Place a sprig of fresh lemon balm leaves underneath your pillow. These will respond to your body heat and release their fragrance during the night.

Though not specific remedies to insomnia, some herbs we use in cooking can also help us relax at night – see Chapter 6 on Food and Drink.

Flower Remedies

These are the bottled essences of flowers and they work primarily on subtle energies such as the emotions, as well as producing physical effects. Take a few drops diluted in a small glass of water before going to bed, and reinforce the remedy by taking it again on waking, and a couple of times during the day.

There are now many different collections of remedies, but one of the first and most easily available is the Bach Flower Remedies that were devised in England by Dr Edward Bach while he explored his local countryside. The range is divided into 7 categories of emotions, including fear, uncertainty, loneliness, and over-sensitivity. It is quite a large range and the following remedies are just a small selection:

Mimulus	for fear of the dark, or of being alone
Rock Rose	for night frights
Hornbeam	a good remedy for overtiredness
Clematis	of use when you are experiencing low energy levels and finding it difficult to wake up in the morning or when you are feeling tired and apathetic during the day
Heather	for feelings of loneliness at night that make you unhappy
Holly	of use when you are unable to sleep because you can't let go of vexed feelings such as anger and jealousy
Chicory	excellent for anxiety, especially for those who can be overly concerned about the welfare of others
Willow	helpful when the weariness of on-going sleep troubles seems to be weighing you down

The Bach Flower Remedies contain alcohol as a preservative. If you do not want to take the alcohol, add a few drops of the remedy to hot water and leave to stand for 3–5 minutes before taking or use it externally by applying it to the wrists or other pulse points.

Acupressure

This is a wonderful method of enhancing the way that energy flows around and through your body. There are certain points on the body where the energy flow is more accessible to touch and we can use these special places to help our body relax and restore its natural balance.

Acupressure is especially good because we can control the amount of pressure we use and the regularity with which we apply it. There are acupressure points all over the body – some are listed below – and you might want to get a map of these energy lines or 'meridians' if you want to explore this practice further. If you are very attuned to the energy of your body, you may find that you are naturally drawn to a certain area which you later find corresponds with a point. Press on each point gently for a second or two and repeat three to five times before moving on.

If you are wary of applying the pressure yourself you can buy small bandages that will do the work for you. These contain small acupressure cones and are designed to be worn around your wrist, pressing gently on a key acupressure point inside each wrist just below your little finger – heart point 7. Rubbing this point gently as part of your bedtime routine will help soothe and relax you.

Another useful point is 'Meeting Mountains', found deep in the valley between your thumb and index finger. You can find it by resting your right thumb and index finger on the 'V' between the thumb and index finger on the back of your left hand. Trace down the line of the bones until you find where they meet. Just in front of this junction is an acupressure point that you can stimulate by gently pressing your thumb and finger together in a pincer movement. After a few moments pull your right thumb and finger all the way out of the 'valley' before letting go and then apply the same technique to the other hand. This greatly enhances elimination and relaxation and will help restore balance to the system if there has been any disruption of sleeping patterns.

The acupressure points on the outside edge of each nostril will also aid relaxation, and are particularly useful if you have had lung congestion, a history of snoring or sleep apnoea (see pp154–59). Find this point by tracing around the outside of your nostril with your little finger, starting at the top edge and then following it out and around. Where the curve of your nostril meets the skin of your face you will notice a small depression in the bone – this is the point. Press the area gently with your little finger making sure the pressure is aimed slightly upward and inward towards the centre of the nose.

Finally, there are two key points on the feet. The first is just around the outside ankle bone on each foot, and the easiest way to find it is to massage the whole area underneath and behind the bone. The second foot point is by the outside edge of the nail on both big toes. You can apply pressure by pressing down on the outside edge of the nail itself or use your thumb to press down on the point.

If you are wearing the acupressure appliance, wear it for six nights, then on alternate nights, by which time your normal sleep pattern should have re-established itself. If you are applying the pressure yourself, trust your own judgement and sense of timing. It may feel appropriate to work for longer than six nights because the stimulation is not as constant as that of a bandage. Alternatively, you may be getting better results from connecting with the point more naturally. Everyone is different and part of the appeal of natural methods such as this is that you will find your own way. Never use more pressure than feels totally comfortable – think of this as embracing your own energy rather than wanting to impact physically upon it.

Tissue Salts

Although tissue salts are not specifically designed to cure insomnia, they can be remarkably effective in treating this by directly addressing and relieving contributory ailments. If you have not taken tissue salts before, follow these guidelines:

- Don't touch them with your hands (they are delicately balanced). Decant the required dose into the lid of the container or onto a spoon and then put them directly into your mouth.
- Do not take them within 20 minutes of eating or drinking anything strong like peppermint tea or coffee (what are you doing drinking coffee anyway?).
- Very occasionally the symptoms go through a

noticeable 'blip', seeming to become worse for a short time when you take the right remedy. Do not worry if this happens but do stop taking the salts if the symptoms continue for a longer period.

There are 12 individual salts, and 18 composite salts to meet a whole range of individual needs. They are known by their abbreviated Latin names. Those that you may find useful include:

- Calc. Phos. (calcium phosphate) – to aid in convalescence and of use when your energy levels are low.
- Ferr. Phos. (iron phosphate) – increases oxygen transport and energy levels. Especially useful as we age.
- Kali. Phos. (potassium phosphate) – a nutrient for nerves and a general relaxant. Invaluable for fretfulness and nervous headaches.
- Mag. Phos. (magnesium phosphate) – a good muscle relaxant.

Emergency Measures

This is the most unusual remedy of all. It brings enormous satisfaction because it uses the notion of contrasting opposites to bring about a positive outcome. If you must get to sleep and cannot, try this for *one night only* – it is not to be repeated more than once a month. Make a large mug of black coffee, and another large mug of camomile tea. Take them to bed with you. Lie down and relax and do some deep breathing or another relaxation exercise for a few minutes, to allow the drinks to cool slightly. Drink about a quarter of the coffee. Wait a few moments and then drink the same amount of the camomile tea. After another minute or two, have some more coffee, and then some more camomile tea. The combination of the stimulant in the coffee and the calming effect of the camomile seems to knock the body out completely. This is not a good thing but may be less harmful than pharmaceuticals as a one-off emergency measure.

Other Sleeping Aids

There are a vast number of products designed to help you sleep well, from white noise machines, which will mask any background sounds, to mattress toppers and special pillows to ensure your spine is properly aligned through the night (see p34). Many of these are optional extras that are useful if you face specific problems but they do not replace the need to address the basics. Two of the most fundamental factors that influence sleep are your diet and the ambience of your bedroom. If you have eaten a meal that stimulates rather than relaxes and are surrounded by a bedroom full of clutter, even the most sophisticated sleep aid is unlikely to help you nod off!

Chapter 6 – Food and Drink

When we are basically healthy, the mind and body work together to ensure that daytime activity is balanced with night-time calm and quality sleep. A good diet that is rich in variety and contains plenty of different tastes and textures is one of the best ways of ensuring our body is able to function effectively and can deal with all the demands we make of it.

Food can be a cure or a cause of sleep problems. Just eating a large meal or one that contains a large carbohydrate component is liable to make us feel sleepy. Certain foods are naturally soporific – lettuce is very soothing, while nutmeg is a age-old remedy for insomnia. Being malnourished is a very real cause of sleep problems and, despite our relative wealth in the West, there are still a surprisingly large number of people with deficiencies in specific vitamins and minerals. A deficit of vitamins A, C and E, magnesium, manganese and iron is very common in women because we lose large amounts with each monthly period. Eating plenty of raw vegetables is a good way to top up magnesium levels and thereby ease period cramps and other muscle soreness.

Eating late at night will keep us awake, while going to bed hungry will prevent us from sleeping well. Certain foods are better eaten earlier in the day while others help our body to relax in the evening. On top of that, we have our own particular strengths and weaknesses and may find that some foods exacerbate health problems such as asthma or snoring. It is important that you take the time to examine your health history and that of your family, so that you can devise a diet suited to your own unique combination of needs.

When You Eat

When you eat is every bit as important as what you eat in terms of improving or interfering with sleep – the later in the day you leave it, the more likely it is to impinge on your sleeping pattern. Your system needs time to digest food, so you should leave at least two hours between eating a meal and going to bed. This is especially true during pregnancy, if you are overweight, have a hiatus hernia or experience night-time indigestion or acid reflux. You cannot sleep well with a full stomach, and some foods that are challenging to digest, such as pickles and fried and fatty foods, take much longer to deal with, so are best eaten earlier in the day.

Protein is an essential part of our diet but it also boosts our energy levels so consider eating protein-rich foods such as tofu, fish and meat at lunchtime. The best evening meal is one that contains a lot of slow-release carbohydrates, as these make us feel sleepy and deliver energy to the bloodstream gradually, unlike the instant hit we get from foods such as refined sugar. Good examples are rice and other grains, potatoes and vegetables such as corn.

What to Avoid

Certain foods will overstimulate us and we do not respond well to having them too close to bedtime.

Caffeine is an exceptionally strong drug that increases your heart rate and may lead to irregularities, in its beat. It influences a range of physical activities from digestion to the way your muscles work, and can also affect your emotional health, making you feel edgy and irritable. Excess caffeine inhibits the body from absorbing vitamins and minerals so reducing your caffeine intake will not only benefit your sleep, but will also improve your general health.

Caffeine content varies according to the type of coffee you drink, but more than 750 mg a day is not desirable. A cup of filter coffee contains around 250 mg, percolated coffee about 200 mg and instant over 100 mg. A cup of tea contains nearly 100 mg and colas or other soft drinks can contain anything from 300 mg for a small tin (this is especially important when it comes to looking at what we give our children!). A small bar of plain chocolate contains about 250 mg of caffeine.

Caffeine will affect your sleep if you take it after 2–4 p.m. (depending on your bedtime), especially as coffee, tea and cola are all diuretics, making it more likely that you will wake up during the night needing to urinate.

Coffee affects women differently at the various stages of our menstrual cycle. For the first two weeks we are likely to need less caffeine to stimulate us as our energy levels rise, while we are very sensitive to its effects in the second half, the time leading up to our period. If you tend to suffer from cramps, avoid caffeine altogether during the first few days of your period as it constricts blood vessels and can lead to an increase in tension. Any premenstrual cravings for chocolate or coffee may actually be a desire for more energy. Try meeting this need by eating something healthy, preferably carbohydrate-based, every two hours, and scheduling time for extra sleep or a nap. Remember, if you feel tired, the best remedy is sleep.

Sugar is present in just about everything we eat and although it gives us energy we do not need very much to have a balanced diet. Refined or white sugar has no use other than as an immediate and intense energy boost. Too much sugar during the day sets your system reeling along a path of energy peaks and sudden deep troughs, causing considerable disturbance to your system, as well as negatively influencing your ability to fall and stay asleep at night.

The spleen and pancreas are both negatively affected by too much sugar in the diet. These two organs are essential to sugar metabolism (ensuring we have adequate amounts of energy to meet our needs) and to the production of blood cells. Food tonics for these organs include anything that is high in vitamin A and has a yellow pigment, such as corn, squashes, pumpkins, yellow peppers and mango.

If you want to sweeten your night-time drinks, choose a 'buffered' form of sugar such as honey, where the substances that provide energy are contained within cell walls and therefore take longer to access. Natural sugars have added benefits in that they deliver other nutrients, vitamins and minerals into the bloodstream. Black strap molasses is an excellent example, being rich in B vitamins and minerals. Consider reducing the amount of sugar in your diet and switch to unrefined and fruit sugars (that doesn't mean adding sucrose to things, it means choosing a piece of fruit over a chocolate bar!). Start to appreciate the inherent sweetness contained in fruits, cooked onions and rice and uncover a whole new dimension to your meals.

Chemical additives are very difficult for your body to process and eliminate so keeping your food natural and safe is the best option. Certain additives will have an enormous impact on your ability to sleep because they are distinctly unsettling. A few are harmless and can even be good for you – E306 is vitamin E for example – but many have extremely harmful effects, raising blood pressure and cholesterol levels, increasing anxiety, and aggravating digestive disorders. Some E numbers are even considered to be carcinogenic, and have been banned from food in some European countries. These include Es 131, 142, 210–17, 239 and 330.[1] Continued exposure to additives can set up an allergic reaction – either in ourselves or in future generations.

Hyperactive children and those with ADDH (attention deficit disorder/hyperactivity) often respond to the removal of all orange food dyes from the diet. The colourant E150 caramel is suspected of contributing to wind and bloating because of its harmful effect on the digestive tract. It can be found in beer, cola drinks, bread, crisps, pickles, chocolate, soups and a range of ready-cooked meals.

Although the additives permitted for use in food are regulated by legislation, this does not, in this naturopath's view, provide a convincing enough reason to include them in your diet. Legislation differs from country to country and is not consistent. In France, for instance, a large number of E numbers were recently withdrawn from use, and countries as diverse as the United States and Russia have banned many that are still permitted in the UK and Eire. Es 103, 105, 111, 121, 125, 130, 152 and 181 are all forbidden in some countries.

Organically grown foods are more in harmony with

---

1 Taken from a list published by the Hospital Centre of Chaumont, France, based on information provided by the research centre at Villejuif Hospital. Reprinted in *Irish Health Today*, 1 September 2000

the body and cause fewer problems than those that are chemically grown. Avoiding additives, preservatives, E numbers, artificial colourants and other synthetics may be time-consuming, but the pay-off is a healthy body that is better able to function as it should.

Food Cures

Food can provide an immediate answer to specific sleep difficulties. If you feel agitated and over-energised at night, consider avoiding spicy dishes and focus on the addition of cooling foods and herbs throughout the day. Make sure you include fennel bulb and leaf, coriander leaf and seed, and choose salads, cold desserts and cooling drinks.

Cooling foods include: the herb coriander (both leaf and seed), fennel, saffron, anise, mint, lemon balm and rose petals (make sure they haven't been sprayed with chemicals); black raisins, celery, courgettes, peas, aduki and soya beans, coconut, cottage cheese and egg white.

If you find it difficult to get to sleep because of problems digesting food, warm your meals with stimulating spices such as cumin seeds and small amounts of ginger. Eat warm salads and soups, and keep away from iced drinks and desserts. Consider your digestion to be like a furnace – you need to provide it with slow-burning foods. Pouring ice-cubes in will only put the fire out! The amount of work involved in processing iced or previously frozen foods can be enormous, and often results in the food being insufficiently digested. This is also true for supplements and remedies that have been freeze-dried or frozen.

Warming foods include: all animal proteins including fish and egg yolks; chillis, carrots, beetroot, horseradish, onions, peppers, radishes and tomatoes, mustard, garlic, fenugreek and salt, and also citrus fruit, berries, carrots, corn, wheat, sesame seeds and alcohol.

These simple measures can have quite an impact on how ready we feel for sleep, as well as reducing the incidents of disturbed digestion that can impair relaxation. Always remember not to eat a large meal within two hours of your normal bedtime.

Some of the elements present in food directly encourage a good night's sleep. B vitamins help support the nervous system, enhancing both sleep and dream activity. Eat green vegetables, especially broccoli, nuts and seeds, and occasionally eggs and seafood to ensure good levels. Vegetarians need to ensure they get enough Vitamin B_{12} which is present in meat but not many vegetables. It is often added to enriched soya products, margarines and some surprising foods such as breakfast cereals. Other sources include eggs, marmite, dairy foods and many types of fish.

Carbohydrates are comforting and, used wisely, can prevent us from reaching for the instant gratification of sweets when we feel we need an energy boost. The effects of slow-release carbohydrates have already been mentioned and there is much to be said for sticking to regular, planned mealtimes so that we provide the energy our body needs in a systematic way and a sustainable form.

Foods that are rich in the amino acid (protein building block) tryptophan also help induce sleep. These include milk, turkey and tuna fish, along with most carbohydrates. If there is sufficient vitamin B_6 in the body, tryptophan will work with it to produce serotonin, a powerful neurotransmitter that is intimately involved with our sleep/wake patterns. The presence of tryptophan may be part of the reason that a warm, milky drink can be successful in inducing sleep.

Calcium is a mineral that we are all well aware of because of its contribution to healthy teeth and bones, and also because of the decreasing bone density that results from its loss after the menopause. Having adequate levels of calcium in the diet is good preventative medicine, but it can also aid sleep. The mineral works in conjunction with magnesium to help regulate our cardiovascular system, and its presence also enables the release of neurotransmitters, including serotonin, within the brain.

Good sources of calcium include broccoli, oats, millet, sesame seeds and raw vegetables, all of which are better than dairy foods. Kelp and other seaweeds are a great addition to our diet, being rich in minerals and very tasty. Look out for nori sheets which are delicious when toasted and flaked over rice, or nori flakes which can be sprinkled on to soup or risotto just before serving. Carageen can be ground and used as a condiment, or as an ingredient in desserts. Nettles, parsley, chicory, dandelion, watercress and camomile flowers are all high in calcium and deliver it to the body in a form that is easily absorbed. Sesame seeds can be made into the most delicious products including: gomasio, where the seeds are mixed with sea salt to produce a delicious seasoning; halva, which is a wonderful sweet made with honey and nuts; and tahini, the paste which can be spread like peanut butter or used as a dip or to thicken sauces and soups.

All of these are good alternatives to dairy products, which can contribute to sleep problems by encouraging the production of mucus, as can wheat. Those who suffer from mucus congestion will know how difficult it is to sleep when breathing is difficult or when the chest is congested, and even a simple cold will respond well to the reduction of mucus-forming foods, especially in the second half of the day (see also Dealing with Allergies p91).

Adding sources of plant oestrogen to the diet can help alleviate menopausal symptoms including hot flushes and the need to urinate frequently during the night (another classic symptom of falling oestrogen levels).

Oestrogen-rich foods include: sprouted seeds (useful for their protein content too), whole grains (in moderate amounts – post-menopause these need to be watched in case they interfere with calcium absorption), bananas, oats, alfalfa, celery, anise, fenugreek, sage, calendula, fennel, liquorice and ginseng.

Supplements

To ensure optimum levels of well-being, you might consider supplementing your diet so that you can be sure you are getting sufficient amounts of the nutrients that assist sleep. It is not advisable to choose individual vitamins, especially B vitamins, without professional advice because vitamins, minerals and trace elements all work together in the body, so taking a large amount of one may throw your whole system off balance. The best way of obtaining the right blend is to take a multivitamin and mineral complex.

Choose one that is as free as possible from sugars, flavourings, colourings and other additives, applying the same care in reading the label of your vitamin pot as you would when choosing food. Producing vitamins and minerals naturally, rather than synthesising them, is expensive and you tend to get what you pay for. Let your practitioner guide you, or shop around. If possible choose a supplement that is hypoallergenic and uses non-gelatine capsules or natural tabletting ingredients – this will always be mentioned on the label.

Tryptophan and melatonin can both be taken as a supplement, but they are not licensed for use in Europe. One sleep aid that is currently available, however, is 5HTP – a nutritional supplement that helps 'build' the neurotransmitter seratonin.

Don't take general supplements for ever – use them as a support for your diet and always have seasonal breaks. You are most likely to need them during the winter months, when you have been ill or when you are stressed.

Relaxing Herbs

Herbs are incredibly versatile. We have already looked at how they can be used as a remedy for insomnia and in aromatherapy but they also taste good too! Adding herbs to your meals enables you to benefit from both their flavour and their medicinal effects.

Here is a selection of some of the more relaxing herbs that can be added to meals or made into tea. You may find others that work well for you, including aniseed, lime flowers or linden blossom, vervain and hops.

Basil is a wonderfully peppery herb with a strong flavour that is used frequently in Italian cooking. It tones the nervous system and is a natural tranquilliser. You can grow basil easily on your window sill. Add a few leaves to salad or to a sandwich.

Borage is a beautiful plant with delightful blue star-shaped flowers. These can be added to summer-time drinks, or the leaves, which have a fine, cucumber-like flavour, can be chopped and added to salads. Borage is a very rich source of GLA (gamma linoleic acid, a wonderful substance that has a regulatory effect on the hormones, the menstrual cycle, cramping and other symptoms associated with PMT), containing more than evening primrose. It is also an antidepressant.

Camomile is one of the best-known relaxing herbs and is especially beneficial to digestion. It is also a good anti-inflammatory, which makes it great for treating period cramps. Use the dried or fresh flowers for tea and add a slice of lime or lemon. You should not use camomile every day, however, because you can overdose on it and overstimulate your digestion rather than relaxing it.

Dill is also soothing to the digestion (it was the original gripe water) and its name comes from the Anglo-Saxon word meaning to lull or soothe. It facilitates sleep and relieves gas and indigestion too. Make a tea from dill seeds and take once a day.

Lemon balm, also called melissa, calms nervous tension and soothes indigestion. The leaves from this wonderfully aromatic plant make a pleasant tea or you can just pick them and leave them fresh in a pot-pourri to scent your bedroom. If crushed on the forehead they will relieve a tension headache as well as relaxing you enough to enable you to sleep. To take lemon balm as a tea, use 3 fresh leaves per mug of water and take up to twice a day.

Lemon verbena has a similar but more powerful flavour and is a strong sedative. You can buy lemon verbena teabags but make sure you note the instructions on how long to leave the bag steeping. Or you can grow the plant yourself and add 1 leaf to a cup of hot water to be taken once a day.

Mint – this prolific little herb is good if you feel agitated. Cram a teapot full of the fresh leaves and infuse in boiling water for 3–5 minutes for a delicious tea that will also aid digestion. Choose different varieties to vary the flavour – from apple mint to eau-de-cologne and Moroccan mint (this is especially good for tea). Take up to twice a day in warmer weather. If you drink mint tea regularly, do make it weaker – about one-third the normal strength.

Oregano is a powerful sedative, and tastes wonderful in Italian or Mediterranean cooking. This or marjoram can be added to every meal and both have the added benefit of stimulating the immune system. Both are good remedies for chest infections.

Sage is a powerful tonic that can be useful when we are suffering from stress or nervous exhaustion. This familiar herb can be made into a tea or added to meals. The leaves have a distinctive taste, so do not be too liberal with them! When making tea, use 2 fresh leaves to a pot and infuse for just 1 minute. Do not take more than once a day.

Sweet cicely is relaxing and aids digestion. It also relieves flatulence. You can enjoy the mild aniseed flavour of the young fruit or chop the leaves into soups or salads. When you are stewing fruit, add a few sprigs of this herb to the dish and you will need less sugar.

Of course herbs are not the only thing that can enhance our menu. Flowers such as geranium and rose impart their own special benefits to a meal. Choose rose petals for their calming effect and their work as a uterine tonic or nasturtiums, which add a peppery taste to any salad and are rich in minerals.

Dealing with Allergies

Even if you are careful about the quality of the foods you choose, you may still encounter difficulty with sensitivities or allergies. If you suspect you have a problem with a particular food or food group, try keeping a diet diary. Note down everything you eat and drink, together with the time of day, every day for a month. Mark down how well you sleep, how easy it is to get off to sleep, whether you wake during the night and how refreshed you feel in the morning. You might also like to record any other complaints or illnesses and how they change through the month, together with where you are in your menstrual cycle. At the end of the month, check to see if there is any obvious connection between your interrupted sleep and the food you have been eating.

If you identify any specific foods that seem to trouble you, leave them out of your diet for the next month and see if you notice any changes. Do not give up more than three foods at a time without the advice of your healthcare practitioner, as this could set up a nutritional imbalance. When you eliminate something from your diet, make sure that you are getting enough vitamins and minerals elsewhere.

The most common causes of disruption are wheat, dairy products, synthetic additives and salicylates (see below). We tend to eat too much of these in the West, often in a form that bears little resemblance to the original substance. When foods enter the body bound to chemical additives, pesticides, fungicides and other treatments, our system may not recognise them and can treat them as toxins. The chemical structure of these foods can also be hard for the body to deal with and the size and shape of both the protein and the fat molecules can cause digestive problems.

Wheat is present in a number of things – breakfast cereals, cakes, buns, biscuits and bread – and dairy products such as milk, cheese, cream and yoghurt form a considerable part of our diet. Fortunately, it is now easy to substitute these with mixed grains such as rye, oats and rice, and dairy alternatives such as goat's and sheep's milk products, and of course soya, oat and rice 'milks'. Even if you aren't particularly allergic to wheat or dairy food, reducing your intake is usually beneficial and encourages you to widen your diet.

Avoiding synthetics is as easy as reading the labels,

but it can involve a major change in lifestyle as you cut out all manner of processed foods and spend more time preparing fresh produce. It can also be more expensive to buy organic food but the benefits to our health far outweigh the extra cost.

Salicylates are substances that occur naturally in all plants to protect them from bacteria and pests. When we eat fruit or vegetables, the salicylates are usually destroyed by our digestive process and the liver, but some people, especially children, are sensitive to them and become allergic to foods that contain a large amount. These are just a few foods that contain salicylates but, as amounts are difficult to quantify, you may find that you tolerate some more easily than others:

almonds, apples, apricots, black- goose- rasp- and strawberries, cherries, currants, grapes, raisins and all their products, nectarines, oranges, peaches, plums and prunes, tomatoes and all tomato products, and cucumbers (including pickled).

As they possess anti-inflammatory and analgesic properties, salicylates are also present in many different types of medication. If you suspect you have this allergy, it is advisable to avoid aspirin and aspirin-related medications such as ibuprofen, and to check the labels of all other pain-killers, cold cures, cough remedies and antihistamines. You should also consult your naturopath or healthcare practitioner.

Recreational Drugs

These days we hardly consider alcohol and cigarettes to be recreational drugs, yet they have a strong effect on the body and a direct influence on the stages of our natural sleep and dreaming.

Alcohol may make you feel sleepy but it damages the quality of your sleep because it sedates the central nervous system, making you wake more frequently during the night, often with a racing heart. It is also a diuretic, which means you are more likely to have to get up in order to empty your bladder.

If you have more than two drinks, you are likely to prolong the early stages of sleep and reduce the amount of REM sleep that you get that night. Alcohol is treated like a poison in the body and, although its effects may feel pleasurable, your body uses up a great deal of energy dealing with it. One of the best ways to aid recovery is to make sure you get an extra hour's sleep. To do this, you may need to stop drinking quite early in the evening or make sure that you get a lie in the next day. Your body is also more able to cope with its effects if you are well rested – having one alcoholic drink after only six hours of sleep can have the same effect as having six alcoholic drinks after eight hours sleep!

It is best to restrict alcohol to one glass of beer or wine per day for women and two for men. Although much has been made of the health benefits of drinking wine, this is mostly only applicable to post-menopausal women, and many of the same benefits can be gained from drinking a glass of grape juice instead. One glass of alcohol with dinner may be relaxing and will aid digestion, but drinking without food is not a good idea.

If you smoke you will be disrupting your normal sleep cycle. Nicotine is a stimulant and sets up an oxygen debt in the body, contributing to problems such as sleep apnoea, snoring and breathing difficulties (see pp154–59). It is also likely to extend the sleep latency period, reduce the amount of time you sleep for and reduce your REM sleep. Quitting cigarettes is one of the best things you can do to improve your health. At the very least, make sure that you do not smoke within an hour of sleeping or after waking and never smoke in bed or near children.

Although this is an area that has not been fully researched, marijuana tends to have a strong influence on relaxation and dreaming, positively influencing our ability to fall asleep, but negatively impacting on the quality of sleep and dreaming. It can also lead to increased anxiety and other concerns such as short-term memory loss.

Nightcaps

And I don't mean alcohol! Cow's milk is rich in tryptophan, which is very good at helping you get off to sleep. If you have a tendency to suffer from mucus complaints, soya milk may be a better choice and is also a rich source of calcium and pre-oestrogens. For variety, you might consider using goat's or sheep's milk, or one of the grain-based alternatives such as oat or rice 'milk'. Honey has always been linked with good sleep, but you could try maple syrup, raw cane sugar, brown rice syrup or date syrup. Black strap molasses is another good choice but its strong flavour means you need to use a much smaller spoon.

Recipes

Sweet Milk

Warm 1 cup of milk until it almost boils. Stir with a cinnamon stick, or add 1/2 a teaspoon of powdered cinnamon and sweeten with a spoonful of honey.

Warming Milk

Heat equal amounts of milk and water with a cardamom pod that you have broken open. Pour the warm milk into a cup and add 1/2 a teaspoon of powdered cinnamon and a pinch of powdered ginger. Add honey to taste.

Soothing Milk

Simmer 1 cup of milk with 1 of water and a 1/4 of a teaspoon each of cardamom, powdered ginger, cloves and caraway seeds, for about 15 minutes. Strain and drink while warm. This is lovely for settling the system.

Sleepy Milk

Boil 1 cup of milk, reduce the heat and stir in 1/2 a teaspoon of nutmeg (freshly grated if possible). Simmer for 5 minutes then strain and drink straight away.

After Dinner Milk

Boil 1 cup of milk and 1 cup of water. Place a teaspoon of decaffeinated instant coffee or coffee substitute into a cup with a pinch of powdered clove, cardamom or cinnamon and 1/4 of a teaspoon of powdered ginger. Pour in the warmed milk and water and add honey to taste.

Chapter 7 – Your Bedroom

We all deserve to have a bedroom that is an oasis of calm – a place where we can fully relax and wind down to sleep. We spend a lot of time in this special room and it is sometimes the only space in which we can truly be alone with our thoughts and feelings. The bedroom is where we experience intimacy and sex, somewhere we can be ourselves and let go of the 'armour' we carry in the outside world. In our bedroom we nurture our body and our inner self. We also become vulnerable as we sleep, so it must be a place in which we feel safe and secure.

It is a good idea to dedicate your bedroom to relaxation and sleep, and to remove anything that might interfere with these two aims. This means getting rid of clutter, taking out the TV, and making sure you store your computer in a separate room or behind a screen so that you are not looking at it as you lie in bed each night. As far as possible, try to ensure that your bedroom is a haven rather than doubling as an office or a storeroom. It does not make for a happy life if the first and last things you see each day are a pile of work assignments, ironing and dirty laundry!

Changing Your Bedroom

Making your bedroom a calmer, more restful place needn't require an expensive overhaul – simply banishing clutter and work-related items, and changing the lighting and curtains will make an enormous difference. If some things cannot be altered completely – perhaps your partner needs light to read by long after you are ready for sleep – then do what you can, such as buying them a low radiance lamp that can be clipped on to a book.

The ideal temperature for your bedroom is around 65°F. Essentially the room should be slightly cool but not cold, and some people like to leave a window open. If you are lying in a draught it will not be good for your health, but a cooling breeze can make warm weather more manageable and a room less stuffy. If you experience hay fever, do not open your windows in the early evening and morning when pollen levels are at their highest.

Beyond ensuring the restfulness of your room, you need to think about the quality and comfort of your bed and the safety of your bedding. One of the most common causes of poor sleep is breathing difficulty, and sensitivity to dust and dust mites is often implicated (see p106).

Simple measures in the bedroom can make a world of difference:

- Turn your alarm clock so that it faces away from you. If you cannot get off to sleep, or you wake in the night, you will not see the time and worry.
- Keep your room as quiet as possible – get extra glazing on the windows to dampen noise from the street and consider having the room soundproofed if you have raucous neighbours.
- Use heavy curtains or blinds so that your bedroom is dark at night. One common cause of light or interrupted sleep is that the bedroom is not dark enough and the body thinks that morning has already come.
- Move the TV out of the bedroom. This is easier than having to make all those good resolutions about not falling asleep watching it – and then falling asleep watching it.
- Have a lock on your door. Even if you never use it, it will help you feel more secure.
- Keep your journal or a notebook by the bed so that you can record your dreams and note down anything that is running through your mind and preventing you from falling asleep.
- Keep clutter to a minimum. If you store a lot of things in your bedroom, keep them in cupboards or a wardrobe and cover open shelves with a simple blind so that the room looks calm and ordered.
- Make sure your bed is good, supportive and

comfortable, and that your bedding is suitable and safe (see below).

Bedroom Furniture

The major piece of furniture in your room is your bed, and this should be firm enough to support you without being so hard that it is uncomfortable. The mattress should not sag, but should spring back into place when you move. We spend up to a third of our lives in bed, sometimes slightly more, and over a lifetime that can mean around 222,000 hours. We tend to change position up to 60 times a night, which makes for a lot of wear and tear on the joints if the body is not well supported.

The position you sleep in will influence how comfortable you feel. When you lie on your side, your hips, shoulders and knees should sink into the mattress slightly so that your spine and waist area are supported. Sleeping on your stomach is not advisable because it tends to squash the digestive organs and can lead to neck and spinal strains as the head is always turned to one side. If you snore, try not to sleep on your back because this will only make it worse.

Check that your own bed is as comfortable and supportive as it should be. Lie down and close your eyes. You should feel comfortable and all of your body should be lying on the same plane. If your bottom is sinking into the mattress, or rolling in towards the middle or to one side, it is time to consider buying something new. Find out if the cause of the problem is the mattress or the bed itself.

There are a wide range of beds available, from conventional models with spring mattresses, to futons, water- and airbeds. Consider a bed with a slatted base to allow good all-round ventilation if allergies are a potential concern. These also offer excellent support for the spine – an important consideration for us all. A solid bed with storage space is useful if you want to keep things out of sight, but check your choice for comfort and support before you decide. Never buy a bed or a mattress until you have tried lying down on it, and if you regularly sleep with a partner, check that it suits both of you and that you don't roll together. If your partner is substantially taller or heavier than you, you might want to find a bed with two separate mattresses to accommodate your differing needs.

We don't replace our beds nearly as often as we need to. Cars, washing machines and fridges are all replaced more frequently, and some of us will be sleeping on beds that are nearly as old as we are! No surface is designed to perform consistently for this long. If replacing the bed or mattress is not possible, consider getting a mattress topper. These come in all manner of designs and can make a big difference. I sleep much more comfortably on one that looks like an old-fashioned egg carton, but you can buy toppers filled with air, or foam toppers containing tubes partially filled with heat-reflecting and massaging granules. Once again, try before you buy to make sure that you find one that works for you.

If you suffer from fluid retention, try raising the foot of your bed a few inches off the ground with a couple of old telephone directories, a few planks of wood or some bricks. Raise the head of the bed if you experience breathing difficulties, especially if you suffer from bronchial or sinus problems.

Over the course of a year, you can sweat gallons of water into your bed, so you need to air your mattress and bedding frequently. Pull back the covers on rising each morning and let the fresh air circulate around them. Make sure that you wash your bedding regularly, and turn your mattress over from time to time to equalise any wear. This is especially important if you sleep with a partner, and can stave off the days when you roll together because of the dip in the centre!

Bedding

As with mattress toppers, there are many different types of pillow to choose from and some can feel quite hard or uncomfortable. They are commonly made with one size of person in mind (often a man) and are not always suitable for women. A good pillow should support your neck and head and maintain a straight line through your spine. When you lie on your back, it should fit into the nape of your neck, and when you lie on your side, it should fill the space between your ear and your shoulder.

A common habit is to stack pillows two, three or even four high, and it can take some time to learn to sleep with just one. It is worth persevering, however, as raising your head too high puts a strain on your back and neck. If you are using more than one pillow because of a digestive or breathing concern, try raising the head of the bed instead.

A quality down pillow should last about 10 years, and will be firm enough to spring back when you fold it in half. If you experience allergy problems, polyester or man-made fillings may be more suitable. Fold your pillow in half and put something moderately heavy, like a trainer, on top. If it is flicked off, then the support is good.

A bolster or long pillow is very comforting and can help you feel warmer at night. It is particularly beneficial if you are full breasted, overweight, or pregnant, because it gives valuable support to your body and helps you sleep on your side more easily.

A recent US study showed that 11 per cent of those interviewed never wash their pillows. After a year, it is estimated that a pillow will weigh about 10 per cent more than when you first bought it due to the presence of skin flakes and dust mites. Regular washing at 60 °F and overnight freezing is a good way of keeping your pillows clean and healthy (see below).

If you experience allergies or have sensitive skin, pay particular attention to your choice of bedlinen. Pure fibres such as cotton feel wonderful and reduce the risk of irritation as well as letting your skin breathe. Again, if you experience bronchial troubles, hay fever, dust or other allergies avoid feather-filled duvets. If you prefer the weight of a blanket you may feel better with cotton rather than wool. What you wear to sleep in is also very important not just in terms of the fabric (cotton is cooler while silk is more sensual), but also because of small things like too many buttons or uncomfortable bows. Think of the fairy-tale of the princess and the pea!

Dust and Dust Mites

Many allergies and breathing difficulties can be aggravated by the build-up of dust and dust mites, especially asthma and eczema. Dust mites are especially prevalent in the bedroom, and flourish in the moist, warm conditions of a mattress, where they can feed on the flakes of skin that fall off our bodies while we sleep. If you have any allergies or a dust mite sensitivity, you need to be particularly careful about keeping mites under control. Direct sunlight kills them, so open the curtains and maximise the amount of light you let in. Consider also the humidity of the room in which you sleep and make sure that the atmosphere is not too damp or too dry. Air the room regularly by opening the windows.

Wash bedding and bedlinen regularly at 60°F, and once a month place your pillows and other bedding in a plastic bag and freeze them overnight, just to be sure. If you have bedlinen that would spoil by being washed at such a high temperature, put it in a bag and freeze it for 24 hours before washing it at a lower temperature. Children's toys and teddy bears can also be treated in the same way. You can also buy protective barrier topsheets as well as mattress covers.

To be dust aware means:

- Cover your mattress with a dust-proof barrier
- Vacuum under and behind your bed every week
- Avoid heavy fabrics, including textured wall coverings and padded headboards
- Keep ornaments and other articles to a minimum, or display them in a sealed cabinet
- Choose lino, wood or vinyl as covering for the floor. Buy cotton rugs rather than wool, as these are machine-washable
- Open the windows regularly
- Keep background heating on – don't let condensation build, or humidity rise to more than 50 per cent (install a humidity meter or use a dehumidifier if damp is a problem)
- Wash your bedlinen at 60 °F, or freeze for 24 hours first, then wash at a lower temperature. Choose synthetic fillings rather than down, and cotton rather than wool
- Wash duvets and pillows at least every 3–6 months
- Keep the doors of cupboards, wardrobes and bedside lockers closed so dust cannot work its way inside
- Wipe surfaces regularly with a damp cloth

The Energy of Your Room

Feng Shui

Feng Shui is an ancient Chinese practice that honours the energy that exists and flows around each room of your home. Its basic principles can be combined with common sense to make your bedroom conducive to rest and relaxation.

Do not place your bed under a window, or directly in front of a door if you can avoid it. This makes good sense as it protects you from potential draughts. Also, in many traditions, a corpse would be placed with the feet facing the door, so you might want to avoid this position!

The direction you face while sleeping can influence the quality of your sleep. Some people sleep better if they are lying along a compass point such as north to south or west to east. An easy way to find out which direction suits you is to spend one night in a sleeping bag or duvet on the floor of your room. If you repeat your intention to yourself before you fall asleep, you are likely to waken up pointing in the direction that is right for you.

Don't have a mirror over your bed – this is thought to be too disturbing for the spirit when it leaves your body at night. Whatever your views, it is always good to make sure that you are not troubled by lights or other reflections and that the view from your bed is as harmonious as possible.

You can divide your room into different areas using a basic Feng Shui grid. Place it over a map of your bedroom so that the entrance to your room is always somewhere on the bottom line. It is interesting to see which items you have placed in each area – if you are trying to conceive, for example, you might want to move your bed to the creativity zone. Simply shifting your bed out of a busy area such as the powerful site of the Ancestors may be enough to enhance your sleep

Love	Aspirations	Benefits
Powerful Ancestors	Health	Creativity
Protection	The Way You are Travelling	Good Omens

The entrance to your room will appear on this bottom line somewhere.

Colours

Colours have a very strong effect on us. Usually strong, deep colours are more stimulating than lighter shades which are considered to be calming. Similarly colours from the hot end of the spectrum – red, orange and purple – are more energising and fiery than something from the cooler end such as blue or yellow. Our sense of this, however, is subjective, and some people find that they sleep best in a room that is dark and womb-like. Pinks and greens are considered to be very restful, but this is no good if you hate pink or can't stand green. Look to the natural world for inspiration and consider its effects on you – if you find being near water soothing, then maybe blue would be a good choice for you.

Many belief systems assign specific values or significance to different colours. Within Ayurveda it is thought that green can overstimulate the element of fire in the body, so it should only be used sparingly in a room, especially in a bedroom or relaxation area. Psychics use a colour code to decipher the auras or energies surrounding our bodies. Here green is most often related to the lower part of the body, and is associated with sexuality, creativity and reproduction. Yellow and colours such as apricot and peach are thought to relate to physical energy and courage; pink refers to the heart, feelings and emotions; lilac and mauve to communication; and blue to the mind and thought processes.

If you like a strong colour, try using it in small amounts first to see how well you tolerate it when you are relaxing at night. You could also tone the colour down a few shades to see if this reduces its intensity and makes it gentler on the eye. Avoid busy patterns where possible and make sure that any artwork or ornaments contribute to the harmonious atmosphere of the room.

Getting It Just Right

Indulge your fantasies when deciding upon your bedroom design and decor. Take a few moments now to close your eyes and breathe deeply and easily. Imagine yourself waking up from a long, deep sleep. What sensations do you feel against your skin? Is it silky satin, or the softness of cotton? Can you feel the warm pile of flannel or the snug comfort of a duvet?

What sort of a room can you imagine waking in each morning? What is the first thing you see? Do the colours of the walls and bedding inspire you? Imagine the aromas – a jasmine plant by your window, perhaps, or the lingering heady scent of essential oil?

Enjoy the feelings, sensations and ideas that come to you for a few moments more before opening your eyes. There is every reason to build on your inner desires and plan your bedroom around them. You can start this in small ways – perhaps just changing your bedlinen or altering the colour of the walls. Your body and mind will be telling you what is most restful, so it is well worth listening to your instincts.

Chapter 8 – Dreams

There is still much disagreement about what dreams are and what function they perform. Since pre-historic times, they have been seen as a powerful tool for predicting the future or as messages from a divine or supernatural source. In classical Greece, they were said to provide clues towards finding a cure for illness, and throughout the ages poets, artists and writers have considered dreams to be a great source of creativity and inspiration. The English poet Samuel Taylor Coleridge claimed that his famous poem 'Kubla Khan' was the result of creative thinking in a dream. Today, scientific theories link dreaming to memory while psycho-analysts assert that dreams emanate from the rich stream of the unconscious mind.

Shamanic lore from around the world speaks of the sacred and creative power of our dreams, and how they can transform our waking hours. In societies where these principles are still upheld, great reverence is paid to Shamans and wise women who enter other worlds and levels of awareness when they sleep. Enormous care is taken to ensure that they are always woken gently because of the danger of shocking them from one level of reality to another.

Many belief systems suggest that during sleep the soul or spirit leaves the body and is free to travel – either in this world or in the spiritual realm. This may be the reason why we awake during the night, as the spirit and body are reunited. Maps have been made of astral planes and other realms the spirit is said to visit at night. The recording of 'out of body' experiences has popularised this idea.

Sometimes dreams are interpreted as messages from a divine source or from the spirit world. Both classical and religious literatures are full of references to dreams in which gods or goddesses appear to ordinary mortals and alter the course of events. In pre-Islamic societies, dream divination affected daily life to such an extent that it was formally forbidden by the prophet Muhammad. Psychics, priests, Shamans and mystics all believe that dreams are a gateway between one level of reality and another.

Whatever we believe, our dreams are deeply personal. Sometimes we dream things that we do not have the courage or the ability to act out in our waking lives. At other times, dreams allow us to express negative feelings, such as anger, resentment or fear, that cannot be voiced otherwise. They are formed from the raw material of our emotions, the people we know and the places we visit. As such, our dreams are unique and can tell us much about the workings of our inner life.

When We Dream

Dreams occur in each stage of sleep, but our perception and memory of them differ and although we quite often remember only fragments, the dreams themselves can last for over half an hour. Our night-time reveries are usually very visual but can include sounds and other external input, especially if they occur during a light stage of sleep in which there is a vague awareness of the immediate surroundings.

We are most likely to remember dreams that take place during REM sleep and these tend to be particularly vivid and dramatic. The REM stages of dreaming occur every 90 minutes or so and usually last around 20 minutes, the first occurring between 60–90 minutes after we have fallen asleep. Both medication and sleep problems, such as insomnia, disrupt our sleep patterns, impinging on the onset of REM sleep and our ability to dream. Many of the drugs that are prescribed for depression have this effect, as do some sleeping pills (see Chapter 9).

In scientific tests, 80 per cent of those woken from REM sleep remembered their dreams, while the figure for deep sleep was at most 40 per cent. REM dreams tend to be very detailed with clear, often bizarre storylines and strange leaps in subject or scene. The dreams of sleep stages 1 and 2 are simpler, shorter and have fewer associations than those of REM sleep, while dreams experienced in deep sleep are more diffuse, perhaps focusing on a colour or an emotion.[1]

During REM sleep, the body is almost immobilised from the neck down, but the eyes move rapidly forwards and back. The suggestion is that this partial paralysis might exist to stop us from acting out the vivid events of our dreams.

We also experience dream-like states just as we are falling asleep and before we waken up, known as hypnagogic and hypnapompic reveries. They differ from dreams in that they are less emotional or elaborate. Hypnagogic reveries tend to be semi-lucid, incorporating some conscious thought and fragments of the day's events. We still know comparatively little about hypnapompic reveries but it has been suggested that they might include 'memories' of the night's dreaming.

What We Dream

Sometimes we are just witnesses to the events in our dreams, but at other times we experience very deep emotion and feel thoroughly involved. Whether we are spectator or participant, most dreams seem to fall into one of three main categories:

---

1 JF Pagel, 'Nightmares and Disorders of Dreaming', *American Family Physician*, 1 April 2000

- Mundane, or everyday dreams that appear to be a confused jumble of the day's events, comprised of some of the things we have done and the people we have seen. This may be hypnagogia rather than true dreaming.
- Moving dreams that seem heavy with import, or deeply symbolic. These can feel very realistic and may be pointing us towards feelings or ideas that we cannot express during the day, or aspects of our life that we need to be more conscious of. Another theory is that they are simply a product of REM sleep at its most colourful.
- Messages or snapshots that appear to come from some external, perhaps mystical source or visionary dreams that leave you with a feeling of real certainty about some future event. These dreams might take place in a completely different era, or depict places you have never been and people you have never met.

On occasion we become aware that we are dreaming and seem to be able to influence the outcome of events. Essentially, we appear to have the ability to think clearly and act upon our decisions, although of course we aren't actually moving and the events are only taking place within our mind. This is called lucid dreaming and is considered by some to be another aspect of hypnagogia or hypnapompia, especially as we often wake the moment we realise we are dreaming. These dreams have a luminescent quality that makes them totally memorable and quite distinct from other types of dream. They often seem larger than life, contain tremendous colours or detail, and can feel quite empowering, as we steer the course of events.

There is great interest in lucid dreaming, not least because of what it can teach us about brain function, but also because of its supposed therapeutic value. With expert guidance, you can learn to manipulate your lucid dreaming to explore deep personal issues that your conscious mind can find difficult to confront in any other way. This is an aspect of some psychotherapy and is also employed by psychics and dream counsellors. Although it can take some time and lots of practise, to learn how to use lucid dreams, the techniques are extremely effective and well worth the investment. It is especially useful when dealing with fears and deep-rooted trauma.

Dream Theories

The eminent psychiatrist Sigmund Freud, and many since him, have all maintained that dreams are essential to normal mental health, regulating the psyche by enabling us to resolve inner conflicts and discharge the tensions that have built up during the day. Freud focused on analysing the mixed and often unclear messages that we get from dreams, believing that the 'manifest' content often masked the real meaning of a dream. In order to discover underlying, or repressed wishes, Freud applied a technique called 'free association' in which he encouraged the dreamer to follow the trail of thoughts, feelings and emotions prompted by the symbols in the dream. He believed that dreams allow us to release psychic or unconscious pressure that, if repressed, could lead to neurosis and psychotic episodes. Many of Freud's theories (such as penis envy) are now considered controversial, but his work on dreams and their importance in our lives was groundbreaking.

Carl Gustav Jung was a student of Freud but he disagreed with the idea that dreams were a way of exploring forbidden wishes. Although he acknowledged that the unconscious could harbour repressed feelings, he believed that it was also a source of great wisdom that could compensate for deficiencies in our waking life and help us explore elements of our personality that we neglected. According to this theory, dreams are like gifts springing up from the rich well of knowledge (the collective unconscious), providing us with inspiration and guidance for the future. Jung believed that dreams do not require analysis unless the dreamer often experiences bad moods on waking, but that to review dreams can lead to enrichment of daily life and greater self-awareness.

Gestalt is a humanistic therapy that suggests that the characters and objects in a dream represent an aspect of the dreamer's psyche. If you use a gestalt model to explore your dreams, everything you see will denote an element of yourself that you need to express in some way. Your mother will represent your own mothering principle (your ability to nurture and care); a stranger might represent an element of yourself that you are unfamiliar with; a child could be your innocent and playful nature; and an element in shadow could symbolise parts of yourself that you are not able to relate to fully.

Modern scientific studies have come up with some interesting theories. Researchers at the National Institute of Health in the US scanned the brain and found that during REM sleep the visual cortex and the frontal lobes, which are responsible for integrating information, were shut down. This suggests that the brain is driven by its emotional centres while we sleep. The Nobel Prize-winning scientist Francis Crick proposed that during dreams our brain is 'reverse learning' – going through all the information it has gleaned during the day and selecting what should be filed in memory and what should be forgotten. Added to that is the theory, mentioned in Chapter 1, that our dreams may be involved in fixing memory or learning in place.[3]

Many scientific thinkers support the idea that our dreaming may be purely random, that it is nothing more than the chaotic 'firing' of our neurons, and that we impose our own meaning on it when we waken. This implies that we are selective in our recollection of the night's dreams, and that we subject them to conscious analysis. Further theories suggest that we dream to relieve boredom. While we are asleep the brain rests and recovers from the work of the day, but it does not like being unconscious for such long periods, and seeks stimulation through dreaming.[4]

---

3 See Jill Neimark, 'Night Life (Dreams)', *Psychology Today*, July–August 1998

4 See Ann K Finkbeiner, 'Getting through the Sleep Gate', *The Sciences*, September–October 1998

An expert on dream research, Rosalind Carter, has suggested that dreaming helps stabilise our mood and defuses negative feelings.[5] It can also make matters worse. During depression, we may have sad dreams that exacerbate our mood and many of the drugs that are prescribed for depression knock out dreaming altogether. A psychotherapist might argue that if sad dreams encourage a person to seek therapy, then letting the dreams emerge instead of repressing them might be a good idea.

Dreaming with someone else is a rare but remarkable event. It can take place between people who are sleeping next to each other or those who are a great physical distance apart. Two people may have the same dream simultaneously or might interact with other through the dream. Events like this blast through our understanding and help us appreciate the vast realms of the unknown.

Remembering Dreams

What we remember of our dreams will be influenced by when and how we awake (ie whether we wake from deep sleep or REM sleep), as well as how deeply the dream has affected us. With practice, you will be able to remember more of your dreams and begin to distinguish patterns and recurring themes. This opens your conscious mind to your inner dialogue and makes dreaming a more active and creative part of your life.

---

5 'Night Life (Dreams)' *op. cit.*

To remember your dreams you must first wish to do so, and then find a way to signal this intention to yourself.

- Take some time to think about why you dream, and how dreams could influence your waking life. Put 'dreaming' on your agenda and find out what others have to say about it.
- Choose a journal to record your dreams, as this signals your intention to receive them, and acknowledges them as an important aspect of your life.
- Just before you go to sleep, state your intention to yourself – that you want to remember your dreaming.
- Keep your journal by your bed and record the first thoughts that come into your head as soon as you wake the next morning. Perhaps you will remember a dream, or maybe just a snippet of thought, a feeling, a recollection of form, or an impression of colour. Write whatever comes to mind.
- Repeat this process for at least three days in a row. Soon you should be waking up with memories automatically.

To begin with do not try to analyse what you remember – just record as much as you can, and work on your ability to recall the details. Later you can look back to see if any themes are developing, or analyse how the dreams link into your waking life. You can use a formal technique such as gestalt or be guided by your instinct.

Interpreting Dreams

As already discussed, there are many different schools of thought on the interpretation of dreams, and they differ substantially. Some people like to send their dreams to professional dream interpreters, particularly if the dream is very complex and will respond to being teased out in as many ways as possible. Psychoanalysts and psychotherapists also work with individuals to explore the meanings of their dreams. As with anyone you allow into your inner world, make your choice carefully. Select someone who is experienced and supportive and be sure that you feel comfortable sharing your thoughts with them. The most important thing to remember is that these dreams are yours alone – your experience has coloured them, and your knowledge will inform any analysis more thoroughly than any technique or other person ever can. An outsider may bring their objectivity and distance to your dreams, but the dreamer is still the expert.

If you cannot understand a dream, try writing it down in as much detail as possible, and include any other relevant information such as what is going on in your world, any events that happened the day before or after the dream, and how you are feeling. Then put it in an envelope and set it aside for a short time. There is something magically effective about this technique as it gives you a clarity and objectivity that can throw a whole new light on your experience. Some people find posting the letter to themself particularly effective –

perhaps it is the symbolism of sending the dream away and waiting for its return.

If you are woken in the night by your dreams, there may be a good reason. It is possible that you are being disturbed by some physical event or just happen to be at a point in your sleep cycle when you were close to wakening. However it could be that your inner self is trying to draw your attention to something important. If you have dreams that contain sensations such as choking or suffocating, you may be experiencing sleep apnoea, and you should consider having a health check (see p157). It is a good idea to pay particular attention to dreams that wake you in the night and record them in your journal so that you can work through them in the morning.

There are times when we seem to dream the same dream over and over again, perhaps night after night, or at important moments in our life. This really argues the case for interpreting your dreams and learning what your silent self is trying to bring to your attention. Start with the feelings that are involved because these will always be important. Let yourself stay with any difficult emotions and think about other occasions when you have felt the same way. What comforted you during those times, or what comfort would you have liked to receive? Once you have held the tension of these feelings, you will be able to analyse the events of your dream more dispassionately. It is surprising how much clearer things can become when you begin to acknowledge the emotions that colour them.

Some dreams seem to defy rational explanation. These dreams may be rare, but always leave a lasting impression, so it is worth marking them in a special way. Perhaps there is a theme or motif that you can incorporate into your daily life, making a powerful statement about the bond between your sleeping and waking self.

Familiar Themes

There are dreams and dream elements that are common to us all. This echoes Jung's ideas about the collective unconscious, an instinctive shared wisdom, that can emerge through our dreams. As with all interpretations, what we make of these dreams will depend largely on our own understanding.

Going to the toilet may represent our self-esteem, or indicate that we need to rid ourselves of something unpleasant. Nakedness, especially in public places, can symbolise our sense of vulnerability, a fear of being exposed, or mean that we have something to hide. A lot depends on how we experience the dream – if we find it liberating, then we might enjoy exploring our vulnerability. If our nudity is not noticed by others, our fears may be unfounded.

Falling is another common theme and often occurs in the early stages of sleep, accompanied by twitches and jerks of the body. It might denote our journey into deeper levels of being, or reflect feelings of instability and insecurity. Freud interpreted this type of dream as an indication that the dreamer was about to give in to a sexual urge.

Flying is often associated with a sense of freedom, or with our spiritual self. Flying with ease suggests that you are on top of things, while difficulty staying aloft may mean you are struggling to maintain control. Sitting an exam is another common theme and tells us much about our anxiety levels. Do we understand the questions? Can we give the right answers? Will we pass?

A house may represent the body (our physical home); a car or other means of transport the way we are travelling in our life; water with all its power and energy, the feelings that sustain us, or the emotions that overwhelm us at difficult times.

Being chased in a dream is another symptom of anxiety. The pursuer may represent a part of us that we have become detached from, or difficult feelings that we may have a problem admitting to, such as fear or anger. Dreams of being chased are very common in those who suffer from post-traumatic stress disorder. (See also p145).

There is usually much to be found in our dreams if we go looking. Perhaps the season will be relevant, or the town or city we find ourselves in. If we were last there in our waking life 15 years ago, what was going on then and, equally importantly, how may that be relevant now? It is often the personal detail of the dream that carries as much importance as the big picture. This is where both the sceptics and the professional dream interpreters find common ground. If, as some modern thinkers maintain, the conscious input – our interpretation – is all that matters, then the process is still useful because we will be examining questions we want to raise. It doesn't matter if the material of our dreams is flotsam and jetsam, it is what we make of it that counts. If, on the other hand, our dreams really are the mirror of our unconscious, then they are a great way of getting a closer look! The most powerful associations are always those we make ourselves – so whether a house is supposed to represent your body or your past is immaterial if it has strong connections for you and means something different. Good questions to ask yourself when you seek to interpret your dreams are:

- What emotion is associated with this?
- Does it remind me of anything or anyone?
- Can I recognise a connection to anything else – perhaps an issue I have been wrestling with?
- Is there a pattern here? Is it a relationship or event?
- What comes next? Sometimes the dream does not give us the answer, but leads us towards it so that we can make the final connection in our waking life.

Nightmares

Nightmares are particularly vivid and disturbing and they usually occur on arousal from REM sleep. They are different to night terrors (see p160) in that we have no trouble waking from them and can usually remember the dream. Recurring nightmares are a common symptom of post-traumatic stress disorder and may also be caused by REM sleep deprivation. Nightmares are also one of the major side effects of sleeping pills or can occur as part of withdrawal symptoms (see p138).

Above all, a nightmare might be a strong message that something in your world is not right. It may be that the story of the nightmare can lead you in the right direction, holding clues in the symbols, locations and events that are involved. As with any dream it can be especially useful to note the point at which you awake. Is your nightmare drawing your attention to some special fear or anxiety that you are now ready to address?

Daydreaming

Daydreaming is something we all do when we switch off from reality for a moment, and fantasise about doing something different or being somewhere else. This ability can be harnessed to improve both our waking lives and our night-time sleep. Being a good dreamer means you have strong imaginative skills, and these can be used as a powerful aid to help you achieve your goals.

When you can see something happening in your mind's eye, you are a step closer to experiencing it as reality. The more flesh you add to the image, the stronger and more realistic it will appear. This means embellishing it, extending the scenario, and colouring the whole scene in rich, vibrant detail. When you add emotions and sensations to the picture, you make the whole experience feel much more lifelike. So next time you catch yourself daydreaming, improve and enhance it as much as you can – smell the roses, touch their velvety petals, hear the bees buzzing around you.

Nowadays, to be called a dreamer is often an

indication that we are not practical or adept at implementing our ideas. In fact, the ability to dream can deepen our experience and helps us to make our dreams become a reality.

Chapter 9 – Sleeping Pills

Sleeping pills and sedatives can have a profound effect on our waking life as well as our sleeping habits. In the short term, they may be considered invaluable for dealing with extreme situations, such as the death of a loved one or when we are recovering from shock. They can also help us adjust when we are travelling to new time zones. In the long term, however, they tend to cause as many difficulties as they resolve.

In the National Sleep Foundation poll, 41 per cent of all women surveyed said that they had suffered from insomnia at some point over the preceding year, so it is perhaps not surprising to learn that one in four women over the age of 35 has taken medication to help sleep.[1] Often this is just a temporary measure, using low-dosage sleeping aids that can be bought over

1 http://ww.sleepfoundation.org

the counter, but some people are systematically taking strong drugs every night before they go to bed. Many are unaware of the possible long-term effects or they may think that these drugs are beneficial because they have been prescribed by their doctor.

Sleeping pills are extremely potent. Within four to six weeks, or even sooner, the body develops a tolerance to most varieties, which means that we require ever-increasing doses to achieve the same effect. We can also become dependent on them, as they are addictive and anyone who has a history of addiction to alcohol or other drugs may find them particularly problematic.

Regular use of sleeping pills robs your body of its ability to fall asleep naturally, interferes with your dreaming and can make it hard for us to wake up in the mornings. It can also mean that you don't explore the reasons why you might be experiencing difficulties, preferring the 'quick fix' solution instead. It is much better to explore all the factors that might be influencing your sleep in order to develop a long-term solution. If you can't sleep now because your inner clock has been disrupted, taking sleeping pills is unlikely to help you redress the balance.

Types of Pill

Hypnotics

The list of sleeping pills available is very long, and the following is just a selection of the most common:

CHEMICAL NAME	COMMON BRAND NAMES
Benzodiazepines	
Alprazolam	Lexotan, Xanax
Chlordiazepoxide	Tropium, Librium
Clorazepate	Tranxene
Diazepam	Temsium, Rimapam, Valium
Flunitrazepam	Rohypnol
Flurazepam	Dalmane
Lorazepam	Ativan
Loprazolam	Dormonoct
Lormetazepam	Lormetazepam
Nitrazepam	Remnos, Mogadon, Unisomnia, Somnite
Oxazepam	Oxazepam
Temazepam	Temazepam
Non-benzodiazepines	
Chlormethiazole	Heminevrin
Buspirone Hydrochloride	Buspar
Zolpidem Tartrate	Stilnoct
Zopiclone	Zimovane
Barbiturates	
Amobarbital Sodium	Sodium Amytal
Sutobarbital Sodium	Soneryl
Secobarbital Sodium	Seconal
Amobarbital Sodium and Secobarbital Sodium	Tuinal

Barbiturates were commonly prescribed as sleeping pills throughout the first half of the last century but they work by depressing the central nervous system, so can be very addictive and cause severe withdrawal symptoms. They were gradually replaced by another group of sedatives called benzodiazepines.

Most hypnotics or anxiolytics (generally called sedatives) work by dampening down the normal activity of the brain and will induce sleep when given at night, or relax and sedate the body if taken in a smaller dose during the day. They may help you fall asleep more easily, and you might sleep for longer, but the quality of both your sleep and your dreaming is likely to be affected. Most of these medications interfere with at least one stage of the sleep cycle, and often reduce, increase, or intensify REM sleep, leading to vivid and disturbing dreams.

The effects of sleeping pills can also linger in your system during the day and may impact on your ability to function normally. They are said to impair reaction times, concentration and coordination, with the result that it can be dangerous to drive or operate machinery, especially during the early morning. You may experience increased anxiety, lack of mental clarity, altered body temperature and, in extreme cases, overt hostility and aggression (although adjusting the dose normally reduces this). Sleep medication can also lead to an increase in breathing difficulties, so you should take great care if you have a history of sleep apnoea (see p157) or other health concerns such as asthma, emphysema or bronchitis.

Many of these drugs interfere with the body's absorption of vitamin D, which is important because it influences the way our body uses calcium, the mineral we need to monitor closely as we approach the menopause. Vitamin B_{12} absorption, which is vital to prevent anaemia and to control the regularity and ease of our menstrual cycle, can also be affected.

Sleeping pills do not mix well with alcohol, and their effects can be exaggerated by antihistamines, cold remedies and antidepressants. In time, your body will build up a resistance to the pills, so you will need to take more of them to achieve the desired effect. This is a vicious circle because the more you take, the worse the side effects can become, especially if you have been taking them for a long time, or you are older and your body is less resilient.

It is easy to overdose on sleeping pills, especially if you keep them by your bed – so don't! The effects of an overdose can be life-threatening, especially in the case of small children whose bodies cannot cope with such powerful sedatives.

A new class of drugs, called pyrazolopyrimidines (often prescribed as Zalephlon or Sonata), has recently been developed. These start working very quickly – usually within 30 minutes or so – and can be taken at any time in the night as long as you have 3–4 hours of potential sleep left. They do not appear to disrupt natural sleep patterns, and have a short half-life, which means they are cleared from the circulation quite quickly. They also seem to produce fewer residual effects and withdrawal symptoms than conventional sleeping pills. They are new to the market, however, so their long-terms effects have not yet been documented.

Antidepressant drugs

Antidepressants are sometimes prescribed as an aid to sleeplessness, particularly when depression may be the underlying cause of your insomnia, or when there is concern about the dependency that benzodiazepines can produce. When used as a sleeping pill, antidepressants can have a serious effect on cognitive function throughout the day. The most common drugs include:

CHEMICAL NAME	COMMON BRAND NAMES
Amitriptyline Hydrochloride	Lentizol, Tryptizol, Triptafen
Amoxapine	Asendis
Citalopram	Cipramil
Clomipramine Hydrochloride	Anafranil
Dothiepin Hydrochloride	Prothiaden
Doxepin	Sinequan
Fluoxetine	Prozac
Fluvoxamine Maleate	Faverin
Imipramine Hydrochloride	Tofranil
Isocarboxazid	Isocarboxaid
Lofepramine	Gamanil
Moclobemide	Manerix
Nortriptyline	Allegron, Motipress, Motival
Paroxetine	Seroxat
Phenelzine	Nardil
Sertraline	Lustral
Tranylcypromine	Parnate
Trimipramine	Surmontil

Side effects commonly experienced include fluid retention, constipation, a bad taste in the mouth and constant thirst. Again, these pills do not mix well with alcohol or local anaesthetics, and can react with other medications such as the contraceptive pill, antacids – even those you can get over the counter – and antihistamines.

Antidepressants tend to alter the levels and effectiveness of neurotransmitters such as serotonin and this can impact on our dreams, either suppressing them or causing vivid and frightening nightmares. Drugs commonly known to have such an effect include all tricyclic antidepressants, including Monoamine Oxidase Inhibitors (MAOIs) and Selective Serotonin Reuptake Inhibitors (SSRIs), and centrally acting antihypertensives or 'beta blockers'.

Antihistamines

Some people self-medicate by taking antihistamines, which are available over the counter from your pharmacist, and are known to make you drowsy. As it is not their primary aim, however, antihistamines tend to be quite ineffective in promoting a good night's sleep. The latest antihistamines do not produce drowsiness as they work by inhibiting a different neurotransmitter. As with any medication, prolonged use is not advisable and side effects can include dizziness, blurred vision, headaches and a dry mouth and throat.

If you have been taking sleeping pills for over a month, it is highly advisable that you begin to seek an alternative. Ridding yourself of a dependency may be difficult and painful, especially if you have been using pills for a while. You will need to reduce the dose gradually and make sure your body is supported in a host of other ways, but the benefits to your general health should be well worth the effort.

Stopping Medication

If you want to stop taking your sleep-inducing medication, talk it over with your healthcare practitioner, and plan ahead carefully. Abrupt withdrawal from many drugs, particularly benzodiazepines, can cause confusion, hallucinations, convulsions and even delirium. These symptoms can begin to appear only a few hours after you have missed your normal dose or they may show as much as three weeks later. Other withdrawal symptoms include insomnia, anxiety, loss of appetite, weight loss, tremors, perspiration and tinnitus. A slow, gradual withdrawal gives your mind and body the best possible chance of making a successful transition and should eliminate most of the major side effects.

The usual rate of reduction is about $^{1}/_{10}$ of the dose every fortnight, but it does vary according to the length of time you have been using the drug, which drug you have taken, and your own reactions to it. Even if you have only been taking sleeping pills for a month, you may need as much as three months to wean yourself off them. It can take some time for your natural sleep pattern to re-establish itself, so think about the additional support you may need in order to cope with this period of change. Plan to use relaxation skills, physical exercise, essential oils, herbs and other natural remedies, and minimise your intake of caffeine and alcohol. Seek the guidance of an experienced healthcare practitioner and take the opportunity to have a full health check. If your doctor did not warn you about the problems associated with some brands of pill, they may not be your choice of support on this occasion.

Gradual Transition

This is a very slow and gentle plan that minimises the shock to your system and gently encourages a transition from prescribed medication to no medication, via a short course of natural alternatives. The idea is to break the pattern of addiction by slowly familiarising your body with an alternative remedy and then gradually decrease the dosage until you can fall asleep unaided. Consult with your healthcare practitioner to decide on an alternative remedy that works for you, or experiment with some of the options mentioned earlier such as valerian and passiflora (see pp68 and 69).

If you have been taking sleeping pills for an extended length of time, you may need to repeat each cycle several times before you move on to the next level. Be guided by your instinct and only move on when you feel comfortable.

Cycle	Dosage	Total time
1	night 1 – normal dose night 2 – ½ normal dose plus alternative remedy	2–4 weeks (depending on the length of time you have been on pills)
2	night 1 – normal dose night 2 – ½ normal dose plus alternative remedy night 3 – ½ normal dose plus alternative remedy	1–2 weeks
3	night 1 – normal dose night 2 – ½ normal dose plus alternative remedy night 3 – ½ normal dose plus alternative remedy night 4 – ½ normal dose plus alternative remedy	Repeat cycle twice
4	night 1 – ½ normal dose plus alternative remedy night 2 – ½ normal dose plus alternative remedy night 3 – ½ normal dose plus alternative remedy night 4 – ¼ normal dose plus alternative remedy	Repeat cycle twice
5	night 1 – ½ normal dose plus alternative remedy night 2 – ½ normal dose plus alternative remedy night 3 – ¼ normal dose plus alternative remedy night 4 – ¼ normal dose plus alternative remedy	Repeat cycle twice
6	night 1 – alternative remedy night 2 – ¼ normal dose plus alternative remedy night 3 – ¼ normal dose plus alternative remedy night 4 – ¼ normal dose plus alternative remedy	Repeat 1–2 times
7	night 1 – alternative remedy night 2 – ¼ normal dose plus alternative remedy night 3 – ¼ normal dose plus alternative remedy	Repeat 1–2 times
8	night 1 – alternative remedy night 2 – alternative remedy night 3 – ¼ normal dose plus alternative remedy night 4 – ¼ normal dose plus alternative remedy	Once
9	night 1 – alternative remedy night 2 – alternative remedy night 3 – alternative remedy night 4 – ¼ normal dose plus alternative remedy	Once
10	night 1 – alternative remedy night 2 – alternative remedy night 3 – alternative remedy night 4 – alternative remedy night 5 – ¼ normal dose plus alternative remedy	Once
11	alternative remedy only	Start weaning yourself off this gradually

As with your sleeping medication, reduce the dosage of your alternative remedy slowly, at a pace that feels right for you. Do not worry if your timetable slips a little – it is better to take longer than to push yourself too hard. It is useful, however, to remember just how much time and energy it takes to make this change. Research is still being carried out as to the long-term effects of sleeping tablets, but it is entirely possible that, as with other addictive drugs, once your system has developed a liking for them, it becomes much easier to fall back into a pattern of dependency in the future. So, if you are ever tempted to use them for more than 3–4 days, remember just how difficult it was to come off them the first time round!

Chapter 10 – Problem Solving

Despite all the information that has been gleaned from research, much of what goes on during sleep still remains a mystery. We seem to be capable of weird and wonderful behaviour – from walking, eating or holding a conversation, to more disturbing phenomena such as night terrors.

In general, sleep troubles belong to three main categories – difficulty staying awake, difficulty sleeping, and abnormal sensations or behaviour during sleep. These complaints often go hand in hand, and a person who has trouble staying awake may take a nap during the day, and then have difficulty in getting off to sleep at night, leading to an increased desire to nap during the day, and so on in a vicious circle. Equally someone whose sleep is disturbed by snoring or night sweats is likely to experience trouble staying awake during the day.

If you find it difficult to get to sleep, or do not wake refreshed, then you may be out of synch with your natural cycles. If you have examined all of the possible factors influencing your sleep and can still find no apparent cause, then it is a good idea to have a full health check. Often the information you get from a partner is the first sign that you have a problem that needs to be addressed. Some sleep troubles, such as sleep apnoea and insomnia can be diagnosed relatively easily, and these are explored in the following pages along with some less common sleep disorders.

Tired All the Time

Tiredness that does not respond to increased sleep is a sign that you need extra help. It may point to a nutritional deficiency or a mineral imbalance, so once you have made sure that you really are getting enough sleep, think about the other symptoms you may be experiencing and assess your overall level of health. For example, daytime sleepiness accompanied by irregular periods and hair loss can be a sign of an iron deficiency.

If you do feel tired all the time, it is important that you consult your healthcare practitioner for a professional diagnosis so that you can work out a successful treatment plan. Usually this problem responds very well to natural methods such as dietary change and the use of vitamin supplements, herbs and other remedies. In the short term, take a multi-vitamin and mineral supplement, and consider a tonic such as Floravital or Floradix. Make sure you are getting a balanced diet with plenty of fresh fruit and green leafy vegetables.

There is a recognised medical condition called **hypersomnia** but this differs from simply feeling tired all the time. A person with hypersomnia tends to sleep for a longer period at night and still feels excessively tired during the day. It seems to be the result of disruption to the 'on/off' sleep switches in our brain. Another very rare condition is **Kleine-Levin syndrome**. This is characterised by two to four weeks of excessive sleep, along with a ravenous appetite, and psychotic-like behaviour during waking hours (see also Narcolepsy below).

Insomnia

Insomnia is the most common type of sleep disturbance, affecting up to 30 per cent of the population each year. It is more prevalent among women and the elderly, with over 50 per cent of people aged over 65 reporting difficulties with their sleep.

There are two main types of insomnia – sleep onset insomnia and sleep maintenance insomnia. The former means that you often take more than half an hour to fall asleep, and find it extremely difficult to get back to sleep if you waken during the night. The second describes the insomnia that occurs when you wake very early in the morning and are unable to get back to sleep at all. Of course, we all have problems with our sleep at some point, but if we experience the same difficulties night after night for an extended period, then we may need extra help.

Insomnia, particularly the latter type, is closely associated with depression, as well as being a major symptom of post-traumatic stress disorder. There are many different types of depression, from short-lived episodes when we 'feel down' to more serious clinical depression that can affect every aspect of our life. One in 20 people have suffered from a severe depressive disorder, so it is not an uncommon experience.

The following are the most usual signs of depression. It is quite normal to experience some of these feelings from time to time but you should consider seeking assistance if you have experienced four or more over a period of several weeks, or if you tend to suffer from extended bouts of depression several times a year:

- tiredness throughout the day and general loss of energy
- sadness that feels overwhelming
- loss of self-confidence
- feelings of guilt and worthlessness
- unexplained physical aches and pains
- feelings of helplessness
- nightmares or the inability to dream
- loss of appetite
- excessive crying
- difficulty in concentrating
- the desire to be alone, or to avoid people, even those you know well
- sexual problems or absence of libido
- addictive patterns, such as smoking or drinking more than usual
- lack of pleasure in things you used to enjoy

- negativity and a loss of your sense of humour
- suicidal thoughts
- disturbed sleep patterns.

Major depression reduces the total amount of time we spend asleep, and the amount of deep sleep we experience. It increases the intensity of REM sleep, but decreases overall sleep efficiency. In post-traumatic stress disorder, sleep latency is increased, along with sleep disturbances such as recurring nightmares. Total sleep time is also reduced, with the amount of stage 1 sleep increasing, and the amount of stage 2 sleep decreasing.

Sleep onset insomnia often occurs when we are anxious about going to sleep – we worry so much about not sleeping that we find it impossible to relax and the longer we stay awake, the more frustrated we become. It can be the result of all kinds of anxiety including emotional trauma connected to bedtime, fear or stress.

Causes of Insomnia

Sleep onset insomnia	Sleep maintenance insomnia
Anxiety and tension	Depression
Emotional arousal	Sleep apnoea
Fear of insomnia	Nightmares and other troubles
Disruptive environment	Blood sugar imbalances
Caffeine and alcohol	Drugs and alcohol

Whatever the reason for your insomnia, it is likely to be affected by a whole range of factors, including the various compounds found in food and drink, any medications you take and a host of emotional and psychological variables. Beta blockers, some asthma medications, nasal decongestants and appetite suppressants all contribute to sleep difficulties. On the most simple level, it is hard to get off to sleep if you are feeling uncomfortable physically or emotionally, if you are lonely or if you are troubled by the events of the day. Similarly, it is important to look around you to make sure that you are not waking up in response to some environmental disruption such as noisy neighbours, daylight flooding in, or the movements of your partner.

Although there are few things worse than lying in bed tossing and turning, it is important to take a positive approach to sleeplessness. If you are feeling wide awake, do an internal audit to find out what is going on, or get up and do something peaceful that will take your mind off your worries and help to relax. Go to the kitchen and make yourself a warm drink, get up and read something easy, or go and do whatever is preying on your mind.

We do need to sleep, but it is worth applying some common sense. You aren't going to go mad or lose your hair if you have a bad night and you can always go to bed earlier the next night. Work out what is keeping you awake, and acknowledge that you can do something about it – this should give you the peace of mind you need to relax.

Resetting Your Inner Time Clock

If you routinely get to sleep later than you need to:

- Make sure that you are exposed to maximum

amounts of natural light as soon as you wake up.

- Be ruthless about avoiding stimulants like caffeine and sugar.
- Establish your wind-down routine for the end of the day and stick to it.
- Be prepared to experience some tiredness during this time, but resist the urge to nap.

If your natural schedule is too early for your needs, and you find yourself wanting to go to bed and waking too early, you may be subject to what scientists call advanced sleep phase syndrome.

To lengthen your days:

- Spend as much time as you can in bright natural light during the afternoon or evening.
- Avoid bright light in the early morning as much as possible – keep your bedroom window curtains drawn (you could even consider wearing sunglasses until noon).
- Take late afternoon and early evening strolls, and have your evening meal out of doors when the weather allows.
- Consider wearing earplugs to sleep to keep out the sounds of the early morning

Wake Up Lots in the Night?

One of the most common causes of waking in the night is a full bladder. This can be remedied by not drinking much after 7 p.m. It may also be a sign of hormonal changes, such as the drop in oestrogen levels that occurs as we approach menopause. Have a full health check to make sure there is nothing that requires your attention. Also check that you are not interrupting your sleep through the use of drugs – especially everyday ones such as caffeine, nicotine and alcohol.

Being overweight may cause you discomfort when you turn over in the night, or impact on your breathing during the REM stages of sleep when you rely on your diaphragm, so consider whether this might be what is waking you.

If you sleep with someone it may be worth checking that you are not reacting to some movement on their part, or to their snoring. Some of us are extremely sensitive to changes in the immediate environment, and can be disturbed by something as minor as a neighbour turning on a light or faint noises from the street.

If you wake in the middle of dreaming, it may be that your 'inner self' is trying to bring some aspect of your experience to your attention. Write down as much of the dream as you can, but leave the analysis until the morning!

Perhaps the pattern of your day is not active or regular enough to allow your sleeping rhythms to assert themselves fully. Make sure that you go to bed feeling physically tired and that you have a work/rest pattern that satisfies both mind and body.

Night-time Hunger

However good the advice to give yourself at least two hours between eating and retiring for the night may be, some of us simply need to eat more frequently than others. A drop in blood glucose levels will automatically waken us up as the brain is highly dependent on this sugar.

Take a substantial drink, such as a milk or a soya 'milk' based nightcap (see pp95–7) half an hour before bed time. If this does not fill you up, eat something light such as crackers, fruit or some crispbread. If you still waken at night feeling hungry, increase the amount of food you eat before bed until you reach the stage where you can sleep through the night but do also make sure that you are eating enough during the day. Always have a substantial breakfast and eat regular filling meals and snacks.

If you do wake up in the night, carbohydrates such as cereal bars are good, or you could snack on a piece of fruit. Always sit up when you eat, and do not lie down for at least 10 minutes after you have finished your food.

Occasionally, people have been known to wake up in the kitchen, or en route to the fridge. This is connected more to sleepwalking than to hunger, and is often a sign of stress. If you find yourself in this situation, take whatever steps you can to reduce the stress in your life. Amend your bedtime routine to include some relaxation techniques, and do not let yourself become too over-tired.

Restless Legs or Ekbom's Syndrome

This is a mildly unpleasant creeping sensation in the legs, coupled with a sudden jerk or twitch, or an irresistible urge to move your limbs. It tends to happen during the evening or when you are tired, but is most common when you are just about to fall asleep. It is linked to fatigue and anxiety, and is more prevalent among smokers and those suffering from stress. It can also occur during pregnancy, or as a symptom of serious health concerns such as a stroke or kidney disease.

It is thought that the main cause of Ekbom's syndrome is a reduction in the oxygen received by muscle or nerve cells, which almost always occurs in connection with malabsorption syndromes. It is highly advisable that you consult your healthcare practitioner if you suffer from these sensations regularly, as there are usually other problems associated with poor circulation or lowered nutrition.

Once a full nutritional assessment has been made, this condition may respond well to folic acid and vitamin E supplements. Restless legs can also signal an imbalance in the calcium/magnesium ratio in your body, so consider reducing the amount of salt you take and make sure that you are eating plenty of salads and fresh vegetables. A good remedy is the tissue salt Mag. Phos., or you might consider a balanced calcium and magnesium mineral tablet. Remedies that increase iron levels should help, because this is how oxygen is carried in the blood. Use either a herbal-based liquid such as Floradix or Floravital, or take the tissue salt Ferrum Phos. Consider taking ginkgo biloba to improve overall circulation, or co-enzyme Q (sometimes marketed as CoQ10) to encourage oxygen uptake in the cells. Alcohol and caffeine aggravate the symptoms so switch to herbal teas and reduce your alcohol intake.

It is also recommended that you have a full physical check to make sure that there are no underlying structural problems. Pressure from carrying too much weight, poor abdominal support, or just the effects of time and gravity can cause similar symptoms.

Keeping your feet warm while your legs are cool brings relief to some people, as does ensuring good circulation – make sure you go for a walk each day, and include some gentle foot stretches and leg exercises, such as the ones outlined below:

- Sit on the bed with your calves well supported, and your feet hanging over the edge. Slowly rotate your feet around, making circles first to the right, and then to the left, one foot after the other. These movements should be slow and careful, but the circles should be big enough for you to feel the stretch up into your calves.
- Next make your toes do a Mexican wave, sending a ripple of movement along from one toe to the next and back again.
- Stand up, take hold of one foot and and bring your heel up close to your bottom so that you can feel the stretch down the front of your thigh. Repeat with the other leg.
- Then straighten up and let your upper body reach down towards the ground until you feel a gentle but sure stretch in your hamstrings at the back of each thigh.

- Finish this sequence by sitting back down on the bed and first flexing and then pointing your feet. Hold each stretch for a moment or so.

Keep all your movements slow and fluid. You should not feel any burn or pain, just a gentle stretch.

Beyond coldness in the legs and especially the feet, other symptoms of poor circulation include occasional pins and needles, burning pains, a slow reaction to changes in temperature, chilblains, and feelings of weakness or dizzy spells.

Weight Problems

Those of us who are slightly overweight tend to sleep more easily and for longer than women of average or below average weight. Obesity has a very negative effect on sleep, however, and is a contributing factor in complaints such as sleep apnoea, breathing obstructions and snoring. Following any form of weight-control diet is not a good idea if you are presently experiencing sleep problems as it can interrupt your patterns further, but if you are sleeping well, then it might be a good time to consider your diet and begin taking regular exercise. Eating disorders such as anorexia and bulimia all impact negatively on the quality and quantity of our sleep.

Snoring

This is a distressing complaint that can cause real disruption to your sleep and leave you feeling exhausted.

As you relax at night, the muscles in your tongue, throat and mouth begin to sag and when you breathe the sagging tissues can vibrate, producing the snoring sound we are all familiar with. There are a number of factors that aggravate snoring – a build-up of mucus in the sinuses, nasal polyps, an anatomically extended uvula (the piece of flesh that dangles down at the back of your throat) or even having a large tongue. Being overweight, or taking excessive amounts of alcohol or other muscle relaxants, is almost guaranteed to make you snore.

- Keep your sleeping patterns regular because symptoms are worse if you are tired or sleep-deprived.
- If your snoring is worse when you are lying on your back (this is true of most people), train yourself to sleep on your side. Sew a tennis ball into the back of your nightie or pyjamas and you will soon roll over!
- Keep your sinuses and upper chest clear – cut down on mucus-producing foods such as wheat and dairy products, and make sure that your immune system is in good shape. Consider taking a short course of the herb echinacea every few months.
- Keep your weight down.
- Avoid alcoholic drinks, especially two to three hours before going to sleep.

If you sleep with someone who snores, it can feel as though you are awake for most of the night, but recent studies have shown that on average we lose only about one hour of sleep. The problem is we don't lose this hour in one solid block of time but wake frequently, often interrupting the natural progression from one stage of sleep to another. This means we can miss out on the deep sleep and REM sleep that are so vital to our well-being.

If your partner snores:

- Try to get to sleep before they do – either go to bed first, or ask them to stay awake until you are asleep.
- Make sure your bed is big enough for both of you to roll over and away from each other during the night. The extra few inches can make a difference to the amount of noise you hear.
- Consider wearing earplugs, or masking the noise with a tape of gentle, relaxing music, sounds from nature, or white noise.
- Although you lose intimacy when you sleep apart, it may be worth spending at least two nights a week in separate rooms so that you get some uninterrupted sleep.
- Make sure your partner has a health check to rule out treatable causes.

Sometimes snoring is accompanied by sensations of drowning or suffocation, and it is important that you consider the possibility of sleep apnoea, as this is a very serious concern.

Sleep Apnoea

Sleep apnoea occurs more frequently in women than in men, with as many as 1 in 25 women experiencing it at some point. Sleep apnoea occurs when your breathing reflex is slowed down or stopped for short periods of time while you are asleep. The three main types are:

- Obstructive sleep apnoea – resulting from a blockage in the upper airway
- Central sleep apnoea – primarily found in elderly patients and associated with heart or neurological conditions that affect the ability to breathe
- Central alveolar hypoventilation syndrome – most commonly found in people who are obese, as a result of low blood oxygen levels.

When we sleep, the muscles that keep our airway open relax and the airway narrows. There is normally still enough room for air to pass through, but in some people the airway becomes completely or almost completely blocked. Women experience this condition more often because we have a smaller upper airway. There is a strong link to snoring, and often sufferers will wake spontaneously after a loud snore because their breathing has been interrupted. We may stop breathing for ten seconds or more, during which time the body is starved of oxygen and levels of carbon dioxide in the blood rise. The brain detects this change and briefly wakes us up in order to reactivate normal muscle control.

The characteristic pattern to watch out for is one of loud snoring interspersed with bouts of interrupted breathing that often end in a snort or gasp. Conditions that can aggravate narrowing of the upper airways include:

- enlarged tonsils, adenoids, soft palate, uvula or tongue
- obesity (causing fat deposition around the upper airway)
- facial and mandibular (jawbone) irregularities
- muscle weakness
- pressure from other soft tissues or growths.

The quality of our sleep is greatly impaired when we are repeatedly woken through the night, and there is also the worry that we may not wake quickly enough. This can lead to a range of serious health concerns including heart failure and cardiac arrhythmias. If you suffer from repeated sleep apnoea, you should seek the advice of a healthcare practitioner, because this is a potentially serious and life-threatening condition.

In the meantime, keep yourself as free from mucus as possible – cut cow's dairy products and wheat out of your diet, along with anything else that irritates you or causes congestion. Avoid alcohol for three hours before going to sleep and, if possible, cut it out altogether, along with caffeine, tobacco and sleeping pills. Raise the head of your bed by a few inches with some wood, bricks, or telephone directories and if you are overweight, change your diet and make sure you get plenty of exercise. Learn to sleep on your side by using a pillow as a bolster, or by sewing a tennis ball into the back of your nightie or pyjamas.

You can buy medical devises specifically designed to alleviate this problem. They work by fixing the jaw forward, or holding back the tongue to prevent obstruction. The most common intervention is CPAP – continuous positive airway pressure. This is achieved by wearing a soft plastic mask over the nose while sleeping. A device supplies pressurised air through a flexible tube, and this acts as a splint to prevent the airway from collapsing. It can take some getting used to, but it can save your life.

Night Sweats

You are bound to sweat during the night if you have eaten a spicy meal that evening, or if the weather is hot and humid, but if night sweats occur regularly and independently of your eating or drinking habits, then they could be a sign of other health concerns such as stress or anaemia. Have a full health check to see if your system is functioning as it should.

Night sweats are common during the menopause and can respond well to increasing the amount of phyto-oestrogens in your diet as well as using herbal remedies and cooling essential oils (see pp47–8). Make sure that your room is cool enough and choose cotton nightwear and covers so that your skin can breathe more easily.

When blood oxygen levels are low, adrenalin is released into our system to get things moving, and this can also be a cause of excess sweating at night. Smokers suffer from this condition more frequently than non-smokers or we may experience it when we have spent an evening in a smoke-filled environment.

Night Terrors

Night terrors are a kind of panic attack that takes place during the deepest phases of delta-wave sleep. A person who suffers from night terrors will wake suddenly, possibly with a scream, and may make sudden movements such as jumping out of bed, or running for the door. They may seem terrified, and their heart will be racing, but they will probably return to sleep after only a few minutes and will have no recollection of the episode at all the following day.

Night terrors are most common in children and we tend to experience them less frequently as we mature. In adults they can be associated with lack of sleep, stress, too many stimulants, or with post-traumatic stress disorder. One basic remedy is to make sure we are getting enough sleep each night and to address our habits during the day. Be careful to lower your stress levels and make sure that you go to bed feeling relaxed and calm.

Sleepwalking, Sleeptalking and Other Activities

Most of the unusual behaviour that takes place during sleep is associated with stages 3 and 4 of NREM sleep and tends to occur during the first part of the night.

Sleepwalking and sleeptalking often coincide with night terrors, and the mechanisms that produce them are thought to be similar. One theory is that they stem from a disorder in the way our brain is aroused from slow-wave sleep, resulting in episodes of partial wakening. Most episodes last no more than a few minutes.

Sleepwalking is a very complex behaviour – sometimes we are able to avoid objects and have a sense of direction, although our coordination is often poor. If you sleepwalk take precautions to protect yourself. Move your furniture away from the bed so that you will not bump into it, and place a gate or some other temporary guard by your bedroom door to prevent you from leaving the room.

If you are lashing out at night, you might need to sleep alone for a while to protect your partner, and if you sleep with someone who exhibits violence in their sleep, take great care. There have been cases where people have been killed by their partner acting out violent dreams, so be especially wary if you or your partner use choking, grasping, or focused blows. It is advisable to consult your healthcare practitioner immediately if you experience this behaviour.

Both sleepwalking and sleeptalking are a response to stress, so it is important that we recognise them as danger signals and take immediate action to reduce the pressure in our waking lives. Start to delegate immediately and learn some relaxation skills to enable you to unwind.

Wetting the Bed

This is something that happens to many children, but can be alarming if it occurs when we are grown. It is usually an indication that we cannot rouse ourselves from deep sleep in time to go to the bathroom and may be the result of bladder problems, or as a response to emotional fears and anxieties. If you suffer from sleep apnoea, you may wet the bed as a direct result.

Sometimes women wet the bed after sex, during the night when sex has been particularly vigorous, or if we have fallen asleep soon afterwards. It is always a good idea to get up and urinate as soon as possible after intercourse, as it will help relieve any pressure on the bladder, as well as minimising the risk of cystitis.

If you do wet the bed, don't be embarrassed. Make sure that you consult your healthcare practitioner to rule out any physical problems, and consider having a structural assessment to make sure that your lower back is in good condition. Limit what you drink in the two hours before you go to bed and check that there is no direct stimulus influencing you. A dripping tap nearby, an active water feature, or even noisy plumbing can be a trigger.

Take one cup of yarrow tea each day around noon. Mix 1 teaspoon of the dried herb or 1 tablespoon of the fresh with a mug of boiling water and leave to stand for just 20–30 seconds. Strain, or let the herb sink to the bottom of the mug, and sip while still warm. Take every day for 1 month and then reduce to ½ the dose.

Narcolepsy

Narcolepsy is the irresistible and overwhelming urge to sleep. A person suffering from narcolepsy experiences 'sleep attacks' that usually last for 10–20 minutes and occur frequently throughout the day. The condition is thought to be a result of abnormalities in the sleep regulatory system and is often accompanied by symptoms such as **cataplexy**, sleep paralysis and visual hallucinations on waking and falling asleep. Cataplexy is a sudden loss of muscle tone that can affect just one part of the body, causing the jaw to sag, for example, or the whole body, resulting in total collapse. Cataplectic attacks are often triggered by emotions such as fear, anxiety, excitement or laughter, and they usually only last for a few seconds.

The effects of narcolepsy can be alleviated by scheduling regular naps through the day and ensuring that you get good quality sleep at night, but this is a condition that needs medical attention, so contact your healthcare practitioner immediately if you suffer from sudden sleep attacks over an extended period of time.

Working Shifts

As mentioned in Chapter 2, you have only one biological clock – not one for weekdays and one for weekends – so if you are working shifts, try to keep to that routine at the weekends too. Although this might not be the easiest thing to do and may cause problems in your social and family life, it is the best way to ensure your sleep is as regular and beneficial as possible. You may have to settle for a shorter sleeping 'night' and supplement it with good restful naps during the 'day'. Learning how to power nap is an invaluable tool and will enable you to accommodate other lifestyle needs such as spending time with your partner or your children (see Chapter 2).

- If you are working a rotating shift pattern, try to use the days in between to mould your sleep pattern into the one you will need for the coming week or month.
- Make sure you alter your mealtimes to fit your chosen bedtime and get to know which foods affect your sleep so that you can avoid them when you are under pressure.
- Stay alert at work – use whatever supports are available to keep yourself stimulated and interested. Use stimulants such as caffeine or rousing activity sparingly and wisely. Avoid dangerous situations and make time for your naps.
- Practise deep physical relaxation and meditation to balance your sleep needs.

Jet Lag

Travelling to other time zones can influence our sleep habits as well as our sleep needs. People around the Mediterranean rise early, but eat and go to bed much later than the rest of Europe, for instance, and they tend to have a long mid-afternoon siesta when the sun is too hot to do anything else. When this habit is practised from birth it can be hard to adapt to the sleeping habits of cooler climes.

Alterations to circadian rhythms resulting from jet lag, can be hard to deal with. When our internal clock does not match the world we suddenly find ourselves in, our sleep patterns can suffer severely. We may feel sluggish and lethargic in the mornings but wide awake at night, especially when we travel eastward. Westward travel lengthens the day and brings it closer to our own internal rhythm which is actually set to a 25-hour cycle, but a long journey can still result in increased wakefulness in the early morning and lethargy at night.

Medical research estimates that it takes approximately one day to reverse the sleep deficit incurred by travelling through one time zone. When we disrupt our own sleeping pattern – by having a later than usual bedtime, or a long lie in – the results are the same.

- If you are travelling and are likely to be away for less than three days, it may be worth maintaining your regular, home-time sleep cycle. This can be difficult if you have meetings or appointments, but is less disruptive to you personally. Otherwise, try to keep to what would be your normal sleep and waking times in your new time zone.
- Select a flight that gets you to your destination in the early evening, and stay up until your usual bedtime. If you wake early and then feel the need to sleep during the day, take a short nap in the early afternoon, but no longer than two hours or you will initiate your full night-time sleep cycle.
- Prepare for your trip by getting up and going to bed

a little earlier for several days prior to travelling eastward, and a little later when travelling westward.

- Travel with earplugs and a blindfold to block out unwanted noise and light while you are sleeping.
- Take your own pillow with you if you think it will help, and any other reminders of your usual wind-down routine, including your favourite herbal sachet or essential oils.
- Try to stick to your wind-down routine as much as possible.
- Plan to get outside in the sunlight whenever possible to let the daylight regulate your internal clock.

Herbs and other natural remedies can be useful when your rhythms have been disrupted in this way. Good wake up herbs include peppermint, eucalyptus and rosemary.

Further Help

If you think you might be suffering from one of the more serious sleep conditions, it is important that you seek professional help.

Sleep studies, or **polysomnography**, are used to confirm the diagnosis of a serious sleep disorder. These tests usually take place in a hospital or clinic under medical supervision, and involve all-night recording of eye movements, brainwave patterns, airflow readings from the nose and mouth, thoracic and abdominal wall motion, heart rate, pulse and temperature. Some studies include tests to measure blood oxygen levels (particularly if sleep apnoea is suspected), and acidity levels in the oesophagus.

A Multiple Sleep Latency Test is used to assess daytime sleepiness. The patient is asked to take five brief naps at two-hourly intervals on the day after a good night's sleep. The time taken to fall asleep is measured, together with other readings, such as eye movement and brainwave patterns.

If you are suffering from severe problems affecting your sleep, your GP can refer you to a specialist clinic for these tests, or you can book them privately.

It is also a good idea to consult your healthcare practitioner if you :

- experience any sudden changes in your sleeping pattern that do not seem to be related to events around you, or that do not respond to gentle treatment.
- feel that you are dangerously sleepy without any obvious cause.
- recognise yourself as being seriously sleep deprived over a long period.
- are very worried about your sleep, or the things that happen while you are asleep.
- are tired all the time, whether you sleep well or not.
- are experiencing health problems that are affecting your sleep.

Conclusion – A Balanced Life

When we live a fulfilling life in which we are able to acknowledge and express all aspects of ourselves we enhance the quality of both our sleeping and our waking hours. Some of our needs are obvious – we need to be productive or work in some way that we find rewarding, and we need to balance that with fun and play. We also need to balance the time we spend being sociable or in relationship with others with time for our inner self and more solitary pursuits. We have a basic requirement for movement and physical expression every bit as much as we need to be quiet and still. We must honour that which is sacred in our lives, whatever gives our life meaning and leads us on, and we must also fulfil the practical, pragmatic side of our nature. Then there are our duties towards others and the demands of everyday life. A tall order in a busy day!

A good sense of balance can be found in planning to spend eight hours of your day in sleep, eight hours at work, and eight in service to yourself or others. This is a very broad definition that spans anything from partying with your friends, to relaxing, or exercising – whatever you feel benefits you most!

There is a tremendous liberation of energy when we commit the detail of our lives to routine. Simply following some basic and healthy steps such as always eating breakfast, prioritising mealtimes, and paying attention to our body's needs sets us free to attend to other matters, safe in the knowledge that our physical self is being cared for. And a happy waking body will be a happy sleeping body.

Make an audit of your average week, and see how much time you make available to explore the broad range of your interests and desires. Are there areas that seem to take up too much time and others that are neglected? How fulfilled are you on an emotional, spiritual, physical, creative, sexual and intellectual level? Consider the way you spend your free time – are you making the best use of it or do you find that you waste hours in activites that bring you little satisfaction? Perhaps there are areas of your life you would like to expand on or explore further?

Exercise

One activity that brings us enormous benefits but is often overlooked in a busy life is exercise. Exercise is vital to our health and to our ability to get a good night's sleep, particularly as we grow older. It can also:

- improve heart function – benefits include a lowered heart rate and improvement in the heart's ability to contract
- reduce blood pressure and lower blood cholesterol levels
- reduce levels of adrenaline and noradrenaline produced in response to psychological stress
- improve oxygen and nutrient uptake throughout the body
- heighten self-esteem, enhance mood and help create a better frame of mind
- increase flexibility and strength
- increase endurance, agility and energy levels.

Modern trends towards more sedentary occupations leave us even more in need of good exercise. Even if we are busy, we may not be working all our muscles or getting the aerobic exercise that increases our heart rate and exercises our lungs. Weight-bearing exercises, where we bear our own body weight, are of particular benefit because they work the bones and reduce the risks of osteoporosis – the bone thinning that occurs in response to oestrogen loss during and after the menopause. Walking is the most obvious weight-bearing exercise, and also one of the easiest and possibly most beneficial. Walking up and down hills has a wonderful effect on the muscles of the abdominal wall, improving peristalsis (the way food is moved through the gut) and providing an effective cure for constipation and other symptoms of internal congestion. It can also help relieve period pain. Walking is also free, and we can usually do it when we want and where we want. Where possible do not take your walk along main roads or in other heavily polluted areas, due to the risk posed to your general health by pollutants. There is also little give in paving stones, and this can lead to minor structural injuries to your body. If you have no other option, choose a route that takes you near trees (they improve the oxygen levels in the air), and always wear good walking shoes with additional shock absorbing insoles. Replace your walking shoes regularly, and make sure that you protect the rest of your body too – don't carry a heavy bag and choose a rucksack rather than a bag carried over one shoulder.

You can measure your own heart rate by pressing gently on your jugular vein, just under your chin, with your index and middle finger. As you press lightly in towards the middle of your neck and very slightly upwards, you should be able to feel a strong pulse. Alternatively, you can use the same two fingers to feel for the pulse in your wrist. Make sure you can feel a definite steady rhythm before you start counting. Measure the number of beats you feel for a full 15 seconds and multiply your total by 4 to give you a close estimate of your heart rate per minute.

During exercise your heart rate should ideally be between 60 and 80 per cent of your maximum. To calculate your maximum heart rate, subtract your age from 220. The range for optimum aerobic benefit will fall between 60–80 per cent of this. So if you are aged 40, for example, your maximum rate will be 180 and your training range will be between 108 and 144 beats per minute.

Aim to exercise for at least 20 minutes two or three times a week, as this will speed up your metabolism and alter the rate at which your body burns fat. Exercise is also one of the best ways to handle tension and to get rid of any feelings of frustration that have built up inside you.

The Great Outdoors

We are a part of the natural world, however distanced we may feel from it at times. The cycles and patterns of nature impact upon our lives in very distinct ways and we respond as clearly to the signals of night and day as we do to the changing seasons. In order to keep our inner world in balance, it can benefit us to remember our place within the great scheme of things. We can do this quite simply by looking out of the window, or by spending time outdoors.

Sunlight on our skin activates the production of vitamin D, which is essential to the body's absorbtion of calcium and phosphorus, and therefore to maintaining healthy bones. Looking out at sunlight in the mornings also helps set our internal body clock and watching it set in the evening is a lovely way to mark the end of the day. Our skin is very sensitive to the world around us and delights at the gentle touch of a warm breeze or the frisson of cold, fresh mountain air. Being able to see and feel other growing things reaffirms our links with the natural world. Simply touching some earth with your hands each day is a wonderfully grounding thing to do.

Respecting the changing seasons and the cycles of nature can also help stabilise us when life becomes too demanding. Spending time out of doors has been proven to reduce depression, especially Seasonal Affective Disorder, and can help us get problems in perspective. There is a tremendous restfulness to be found in nature. Just being near water is remarkably peaceful and we can benefit enormously from its calming influence.

If you cannot spend time outside for any reason, try some visualisation exercises. As you shower, imagine you are standing under a wonderful warm waterfall, or close your eyes and imagine that you are lying on a sunny beach with the sound of waves lapping the shore nearby and the gentle heat of the sun warming your body.

A Good Night's Sleep

The best balance to a satisfying day is a good night's sleep. We may define this differently, but we all recognise the wonderful sensation when we waken up feeling rested and renewed, full of energy and enthusiasm for the day ahead. For some of us, a good night's sleep is something we dream of, but find difficult to attain. The advice in this book is all geared towards giving you ideas about how you might achieve a more restful night.

Checklist for a Good Night's Sleep

- Check out your immediate environment – are you feeling comfortable, is the room dark enough and have you got the temperature right?
- Register what is going on in the neighbourhood with your conscious mind so it is less likely to trouble you while you are sleeping.
- Do a body scan – are you feeling comfortable, not hungry or overfull, or perhaps thirsty?
- Do you feel supported by a firm mattress and a low pillow that keeps your spine straight?
- Are you relaxed and ready for sleep, or still stimulated from the evening's activities?
- Is your mind calm and ready to dream or is there anything you need to record before you can relax fully?
- Are you feeling settled and emotionally calm, or are there issues you should consider now that you have some quiet time?
- Are you regulating your time clock and keeping to the same bedtime as much as possible?
- Did you prepare for sleep by establishing a wind-down routine?
- Have you avoided caffeine, alcohol and other drugs?
- Are you physically tired and actually ready for sleep?

Ask yourself these questions and listen to the answers. Give yourself time to hear what your real needs are, and then be prepared to act upon them. Sweep through your body with your imagination and see how you feel – are there areas of physical tension that you still need to relax? To get off to sleep you will need to feel safe and comfortable, and this includes your emotional world. Beyond making your own physical checklist about having locked the doors and the windows, you need to address any emotions that are keeping you from restful sleep.

My mother always used to say 'goodnight darling, have sweet dreams' and I remember the comfort and security that gave me as a child, preparing to face the long journey into the dark on my own. Getting off to sleep, staying asleep, and waking up feeling refreshed all rely on our own unique combination of measures and methods – individually they may seem too silly to mention, but they build into a tapestry that works because they are born of our own unique needs and what we have found to be helpful.

Close your eyes now and use your powers of imagination to help you relax and prepare for sleep. Take a few deep breaths and, as you breathe out, let any tension or wakefulness leave your body. Relax and let your breathing cycle become a little deeper, and a little slower. Notice the sure support of the bed that holds you, and let yourself enjoy the silky smoothness of your sheets, or the warm comfort of the duvet draped around you. Feel yourself sinking slowly and inexorably into the deep sweetness of sleep and dreams, and enjoy the journey.

Resources

Further Reading

Balcombe, BF, *As I See It*, Piatkus Books, 1995

Ball, Nigel and Nick Hough, *The Sleep Solution*, Vermillion, 1998

Carter, Jaine M, *He Works, She Works – Successful Strategies for Working Couples*, Cartercarter.com, 1996

Connelly, Dianne, *Traditional Acupuncture: The Law of the 5 Elements*, Centre for Traditional Acupuncture, Maryland 21044, USA, 1979

D'Adamo, Peter and Catherine Whitney, *Eat Right for your Type*, Putnam, 1998

Davis, Patricia, *Aromatherapy, an A–Z*, CW Daniel and Co, 1988

Gach, Michael Reed, *Acupressure*, Piatkus Books, 1995

Gelb, Douglas J., *An Introduction to Clinical Neurology*, Butterworth-Heinemann,1995
Goodison, Lucy, *The Dreams of Women*, The Women's Press, 1995
Hall, Doriel, *Healing with Meditation*, Gill and Macmillan, 1996
Hird, Vicki, *Perfectly Safe to Eat*, The Women's Press, 2000
The Merck Manual of Diagnosis and Therapy, Merck Research Laboratories, USA, 2000
Northrup, Dr Christiane, *Women's Bodies, Women's Wisdom*, Piatkus Books, 1995
Viagas, Belinda Grant, *Natural Healthcare for Women*, Newleaf, 1999
Viagas, Belinda Grant, *Nature Cure*, Newleaf, 1999
Viagas, Belinda Grant, *Stress: Restoring Balance to Our Lives*, The Women's Press, 2001

Contacts

American Sleep Apnoea Association
2025 Pennsylvania Ave, NW
Washington DC 20006
USA
Tel: 001 202 293 3650
www.nicom.com/-asaa

American Sleep Disorders Association
1610 14th St, NW, Suite 300
Rochester MN 55901
USA
www.asda.org

The British Sleep Foundation
10 Cabot Square
Canary Wharf
London EH11 4QB
Tel: 020 7345 3317
Email: bsf@uk.ogilvypr.com
www.britishsleepfoundation.org.uk

HPRU Sleep Lab
Egerton Road
Guildford
Surrey GU2 5XP

Narcolepsy Network
10921 Reed Hartman Highway
Cincinnati OH 45242
USA
Tel: 001 513 891 3522
Fax: 001 513 891 3836
Email: narnet@aol.com
www.narcolepsynetwork.org

National Centre on Sleep Disorders Research
Two Rockledge Centre, Suite 7024
6701 Rockledge Drive (MSC 7920)
Bethesda MD 20892
USA
Tel: 001 301 435 0199
www. Nhlbi.nih.gov/nhlbi/nhlbi.htm

The National Sleep Foundation (US)
1522 K Street, NW, Suite 500
Washington DC 20005
USA
Tel: 001 202 347 3471
Fax: 001 202 347 3472
www.sleepfoundation.org

Sleep Apnoea Trust
7 Bailey Close
High Wycombe HP13 6QA
Tel: 01494 527772
www.sleepmatters.org

The Sleep Disorder Clinic
98 Harley Street
London W1
Tel: 020 7629 8304
and
St James' Building
79 Oxford Street
Manchester M1 6EJ
Tel: 0161 236 0930

Sleep Research Centre
Loughborough University
Loughborough
Leicester LE11 3TU
Tel: 01509 228480
Email: SleepResearch@lboro.ac.uk
www.lboro.ac.uk/departments/hu/groups/sleep

The Snoring and Sleep Apnoea Clinic
Princess Gate Hospital
42–52 Nottingham Place
London W1V 5NY
Tel: 020 7486 1234
Fax: 020 7908 2492

For details of Belinda's confidential postal Advice Service, or a timetable of her natural healthcare events, or to purchase a Bioflow electromagnetic device for personal wear, contact her at:
PO Box 13386
London NW3 2ZE
England
Email: Belindasres@hotmail.com